FOREWORD BY K~~~~~~~~~~

PUCK STOPS HERE

HOCKEY PLAYERS' HEALTHY EATING HANDBOOK

ROXANNE TUOMELA, AADP

outskirtspress

DENVER, COLORADO

Cover Photo Model: Hayden Kiely.
Front Cover Photo © 2015 Leah Kiely. All rights reserved - used with permission.
Back Cover Photo © 2015 Divine Photography. All rights reserved - used with permission.

Special acknowledgement to Shannon Gilbert for coming up with the book's title.

Outskirts Press, Inc.
http://www.outskirtspress.com

ISBN: 978-1-4787-3849-7

Outskirts Press and the "OP" logo are trademarks belonging to Outskirts Press, Inc.

PRINTED IN THE UNITED STATES OF AMERICA

DISCLAIMERS

Roxanne is not to prescribing or assessing micro- and macronutrient levels; providing health care, medical or nutrition therapy services; or is not diagnosing, treating or curing any disease, condition or other physical or mental ailment of the human body. Rather, Roxanne, as a board certified holistic health coach, is a mentor and guide who has been trained in transformational and holistic health and life coaching to help Readers reach their own health goals by helping Readers devise and implement positive, sustainable lifestyle changes. The Reader understands that Roxanne is not acting in the capacity of a doctor, licensed dietician-nutritionist, psychologist or other licensed or registered professional, and that any advice given by her is not meant to take the place of advice by these professionals. If the Reader is under the care of a health care professional or currently uses prescription medications, the Reader should discuss any dietary changes or potential dietary supplements use with his or her doctor, and should not discontinue any prescription medications without first consulting his or her doctor.

The Reader understands that the information received should not be seen as medical or nursing advice and is not meant to take the place of seeing licensed health professionals.

PERSONAL RESPONSIBILITY AND RELEASE OF HEALTH CARE RELATED CLAIMS

The Reader acknowledges that the Reader takes full responsibility for the Reader's life and well-being, as well as the lives and well-being of the Reader's family and children (where applicable), and all decisions made during and after this book.

The Reader expressly assumes the risks of trying new foods or supplements, and the risks inherent in making lifestyle changes. The Reader releases Roxanne from any and all liability, damages, causes of action, allegations, suits, sums of money, claims and demands whatsoever, in law or equity, which the Reader ever had, now has or will have in the future against Roxanne, arising from the Reader's past, present or future.

To my children, Hayden and Leah,

Without your love, support and faith in me this book would never have been written. You've been patient and understanding when my work never seemed to end, though, together, we have learned how to juggle it all. I am grateful that we experience laughter every day and we say "I love you" several times a day. I am blessed to have two incredibly happy and healthy children. And, please, always remember what great-grandma used to say, "Everyone has their own idea of a good time." If you keep those words of wisdom in the forefront of your mind, you will never judge another. I am proud to be your mother. You make me a better person. Thank you for believing in me.

Work hard. Play hard. Eat well. Give love and receive love. Have faith. Believe in yourself.

I love you with all of my heart,

Mom

In Loving Memory of
Donald A. Gilbert
The Ultimate Hockey Grandpa

FOREWORD
by Keith Primeau

Traditionally I have written forewords on hockey-related books, possibly as an area of knowledge. I have appreciated the requests and enjoyed the opportunity to write down my views or a short story or two as a preamble to some great works. Once again I have been bestowed with the honor of writing a foreword and I appreciate Roxanne's request and will do my best to do her life's passion justice.

There are very few things that I can truly say I am passionate about, not in an obsessively compulsive way, but to the point that these items take precedence in my life. One is family and the other is the sport of hockey. Whether it was as a youth player myself, a professional hockey player, or now as a youth coach involved in hockey on many different levels, as just enjoyment or from a business perspective. If there was one other area that I can reflect on and say I was passionate about, or at least very intuitive with, it would be diet during my playing days.

My intuitiveness did not exist early in my career. Playing junior hockey in Ontario, Canada my pre-game meal consisted of spaghetti-O's and grilled cheese. Not entirely meeting the criteria needed to play at optimal level. As I matured and as my career progressed I became much more acutely aware of my body and because of this I became much more critical of what I put into my body. As a professional athlete, you look for any way possible to find that "edge" over your opponent. Whether it be on-ice conditioning, off-ice conditioning, mental toughness and/or healthy living, any and all advantages become top priority.

As I mentioned earlier, I was committed to knowing what I consumed, but not obsessive compulsive about it either. I tried to stick to a regimen of carbohydrates mostly pre-game and protein overload post game. I also was never big on powders or supplements, because I always felt that if you had a well-balanced diet, your body neither craved nor needed anything else. As the game of hockey has continued to evolve and player development and training continue to re-invent themselves, in this case the sooner the driven and passionate player understands their body and their food intake, the sooner they will have an advantage over their opponent.

My recommendation for this book is to not just read it in its entirety, but to digest the information, draw from the information and periodically review the information. Times are always changing, but one thing stays constant. The individual, who takes care of himself away from the ice, will have a distinct advantage on the ice. Remember your body is a temple; treat it like one.

Thank you,

Keith Primeau
Former Professional Hockey Player

ENDORSEMENTS

"As avid fitness and sports nutrition enthusiasts, my wife, Kristine, and I were very excited to read Roxanne's book. She was able to simplify the science of healthy eating which is by far the most challenging aspect for most people trying to live a healthy lifestyle.

As a youth hockey coach, I find that the majority of young elite athletes do not know how to fuel their bodies properly. And much of that begins with the need to educate their parents. Roxanne's book provides the core principles of sports nutrition. It also provides numerous examples and suggestions for others to follow.

This is a great read for aspiring young athletes and their parents.

Congratulations on your book, Roxanne."

 ~Travis Howe

"As a hockey mom to a growing teen player, I love that this book provides quick reference suggestions for the healthiest (and quickest) solutions to eating around a busy hockey schedule! It also goes beyond and provides the supporting information and specifics for a host of health issues! Awesome go-to book for healthier skaters both now and in the future! Thank you for addressing this ongoing concern for hockey families!"

 ~Shannon Gilbert, Hockey Mom

If you're low on energy, seek out Roxanne; she'll get you back on track. I've never met a person with so much passion and drive to help others. She's scored a Hat Trick with her "Puck Stops Here" nutritional book. Hockey is getting to be so competitive and skilled. Players need to realize that what they are putting into their bodies is equally important as the physical training they are doing. Thanks Roxanne for laying it out in such an easily digestible book form!!

~Lance Pitlick, Former NHLer

"I believe adolescent hockey players, who wish to maximize their performance, will find many practical and useful tips in The Puck Stops Here!"

~Murray Howe, M.D.
Division Head
Sports Medicine Imaging
Toledo Radiological Associates

"Roxanne's book is very informational regarding how to give your body what it needs to perform at a better level regardless of skill level of sport! I learned many things applicable to my own life as well as my clientele!"

~Marissa Campeau, Personal Trainer,
BA Exercise Science

APPRECIATION

Thank you, my dear, reader, for playing hockey, *the* greatest sport on earth. I appreciate *YOU!* Your family appreciates you. Please know that by playing hockey, you have given your mom, dad, siblings, extended family and friends an incredible community with which to share special times. It is a community where someone always has your back. A place where one feels love, safety and belonging. Together, as a community, there is enough enthusiasm to raise the roof off a rink! That kind of energy is powerful, my friend. There are times we experience gut-wrenching laughter and sometimes tears. I will be the first to admit it—hockey and everything that goes along with it can be stressful on occasion, but we have remedies for that . . . Wink! Wink! More importantly, we have memories which we will cherish for a lifetime. Friendships we will embrace forever. I am so grateful for the friends I have made through my son's hockey career. His career has taken us all over the U.S., Canada and even overseas. Be certain that there is nothing more satisfying than being a Hockey Mom other than, perhaps, being a part of a hockey family. It is such an adventure. A real hoot and a holler. A total gas!

Thank you, coaches, for being instrumental in helping my son, Hayden, develop into a united team player and motivating leader. Thank you for inspiring my kid to be the best he can be both on ice and off, as a hockey player and a good citizen. You, coach, are the reason my son loves the game of hockey. And, I thank all of you, all of the coaches' spouses, who have been patient and understanding when your husband was away from home putting in long hours at the rink early in the morning, all afternoon and late into the night—coaching my son on how to become an elite hockey player. Thank you for giving up your husband to coach every weekend and, basically, every holiday for my son's hockey tournaments. I also appreciate that it was often all year long, not just in the fall and winter.

Thank you to all of the team managers for keeping me organized with emails and texts with regard to practices and games and which rink was the right one and when. Thank you for arranging all of our hotel accommodations, restaurant reservations, extracurricular activities for bonding and hired transportation when needed. You made sure all of us—coaches, parents and players—came together to feel the love and build a strong bond as a hockey family, and this, I know, is not an easy feat but you made it happen. Thank you.

Thank you former, present and future professional hockey players for being amazing role models for my son and every youth player out there. You raise the bar when it comes to classy sportsmanship. You exhibit such grace. You are humble. You have great values and you stand behind your morals. The example you set is truly admired.

Thank you to all the members of each and every hockey organization around the world. We appreciate the fact that you see to it and make a point that every child who wants to play hockey gets an opportunity to do so. You do more behind the scenes than people can even fathom.

How many rinks have I been to? I couldn't even begin to count. But I would like to take this opportunity to show appreciation to all of rinks around the world for hosting my son and the teams he has had the privilege to play for. You offer ice time 24/7/365 because you care about the players. Ice rinks are unique and special places. I have personally spent countless hours hanging out in your lobby, cafe or parking lot, so please know, those of you who manage and run the rink, how much I appreciate my home-away-from-home. Some rinks are super cold and, there's no question, I couldn't live without my Uggs® but I do so appreciate a heat lamp overhead from time-to-time, so thank you for attempting to make it more cozy.

I don't believe I have ever had the chance to thank a Zamboni® operator. Please know, I enjoy watching you zip around on an icy patch and never take out a board. It is soothing to watch the ice being resurfaced between periods and I know the players appreciate you and the machine you drive.

Last, but not least, thank you to all of the hotel staff and restaurant servers for making our experience a special one each time we have taken over your establishment. We appreciate your warm and welcoming smile, your hospitality, for simply treating us like one BIG HAPPY FAMILY!

Table of Contents

INTRODUCTION

"The Puck Stops Here"! What exactly does that mean? I am sure you have heard the term "the *buck* stops here," which means for one to take responsibility for oneself, that one's responsibility is not passed on beyond this point. Well, the puck stops here! Today, you are choosing to take responsibility for yourself. I celebrate you for taking responsibility for what you put into your body from this day forward.

Thank you for your trust in me and for picking up this book either for yourself or to help a player whom you love and care so much for. Please embrace the lessons I am going to teach you. These are lessons which you will carry with you for the rest of your life.

What I am about to coach you on is *not* about being on a diet. I ask you to relax and please know that I do not take away the foods and beverages you love. You will simply learn how to crowd out some of the bad and replace those things with wonderful, nutrient-dense foods and beverages.

In the beginning, I want you to keep a food journal so you can keep track of calories, carbs, protein and fats that *you* have and need to consume to perform at your best. By keeping track you will figure out just the right formula for you. You will discover what to eat and when. You will find that the new healthy-habits you adopt will be so easy to sustain. You won't believe how fantastic you will feel inside and out. This is the beginning of *your* transformation. Once you can get on the road to better eating you will rarely find yourself off of the beaten path because you will begin to understand and experience the amazing affects of eating well.

Do you want to make the team this season? Do you truly have the burning desire to make the team? You need to believe and have faith that you are the one who is going to make the team because *you* are going to have specialized knowledge—knowledge which your opponent won't have because you're reading this book. Ask your teammates to get their own copy so together you can CRUSH the other team. *You* are the one others are going to fear out on the ice. *You* are the one scouts are watching and who they are after. *You* are the one about whom folks are going to be asking, "Who is that player?" "Where did he/she get such energy—such speed/endurance, such determination?" "What is going on in his/her mind?" "That player is unstoppable!"

Is your dream to go from pond hockey to playing with the pros? Wouldn't it be spectacular to earn a scholarship? To play Division I? Your journey to stardom starts here and now. Eat well. Eat clean. Nourish your body. Change your unhealthy habits.

How disciplined are you about eating well? If you can eat

well without further guidance by all means go ahead and put this book down. If you need a little guidance, a little push, without feeling like you're getting nagged at (I know, you're sick of hearing it from your mom, dad or coaches) then this book is for you. Please, don't put it down. I want you to find nutrition interesting. I want you to end up *grossed out* by processed foods and things like unnatural ingredients.

You can have an outstanding hockey career but you have to have the burning desire deep within you. You must continue to train diligently on ice and off and nourish your body but what else might you need? A specialized skill. What is your specialized skill out on the ice? Perhaps, your energy and enthusiasm is just what your team needs in the locker room or on the bench. Which skill are you better at than everyone else? Wonderful! Now plan on perfecting it. You've gotta have a plan. Visualize your dream. Can you picture yourself playing as a pro? Now, picture yourself kissing the Stanley Cup. How does that feel? AMAZING! Right!?

So, remember, THE PUCK STOPS HERE! You are in control of what goes into your body. You are taking on the responsibility all by yourself and I am so proud of you. I believe this book will make it easier for you to accomplish your goals. I have thrown in some meal plan ideas and a few recipes. I have provided you with as much information as I can with regard to the nutritional value of some of the healthiest foods and beverages. I have given you suggestions on what you need to pitch from your kitchen pantry. I have spelled out what to avoid and the why.

Please stock your pantry and refrigerator with as many items as you want off of my Recommended Food and Beverage List, included here within. Take it to the grocery store with you and please be willing to try new things.

Now, take a deep breath. You are about to step outside of your comfort zone. You are allowing yourself to be different than others. You are beginning to understand that it is okay to be you. You are ready, I mean, *really* ready to move past your competition. Take another deep breath and embrace the fact this is a very exciting time for you. And may I give you the courage to allow others to stay where they choose to stay in their journey, though I see you as an inspiration and others will want to be successful like you. I applaud you for taking this leap of faith and for wanting to educate yourself on proper nutrition so you can be the elite athlete you so desire to be.

You good? You ready to go? Awesome! Let's get started!

1

DESIRE TO LIVE A HEALTHY LIFE

Some thirty years ago my own desire to live a life filled with joy, happiness and good health began, basically, because over a ten-year span my older brother and I lost all of our family except for a few loving, wonderful and supportive cousins.

Back in 1983, while I was attending Robert Morris College in Chicago, my mom was diagnosed with lung cancer. My mom was a smoker. Throughout my entire twenties I had to watch my mom battle cancer off and on. Cancer first reared its ugly head in my mom's lung, lymph nodes and throat and over time the cancer spread to her spine, brain, eye and then it finally settled in her liver; that was the end of her battle. She was too young; she was only 57 when she died.

Only a year and half after my mom died, my dad died. Tragically, he battled alcoholism. My brother and I were left as orphans. After attending funeral after funeral, I vowed to live a long, happy, healthy life.

I began by understanding which foods were best for me. I journaled my findings, and to this day I refer back to those diaries if I find myself getting off track.

I set a goal to run my first marathon; mind you this item on my bucket list of healthy living didn't happen until I was in my forties. It was the MORE Marathon and took place in Central Park, in New York City; it was magical! I didn't stop running there. After that first marathon, I have since run and walked several more. One of the things I like to do is to participate in a worthy cause, such as a breast cancer walk/run. By signing yourself up for a specific cause you will be motivated to train, to do your best and to not give up on your goal. Between your hockey seasons you might want to consider doing the same and get your family and friends involved too.

I, personally, head to the gym as many times as I can in a week and I also work out with a private trainer when possible.

Taking care of ourselves is the least selfish thing in the world we can do for our loved ones. Please understand how important it is to allow yourself time for self care. Encourage your parents, grandparents, siblings, teammates and friends to do the same. Show support when your mom or dad takes time to go to the gym. Get everyone on the bandwagon to take good care of themselves.

Beyond marathons and working out, I had the burning desire to become better educated on the effects of foods and beverages on my own body. Thus, I attended IIN, the Institute of Integrative Nutrition and became a board certified holistic health coach.

You see, once you set a goal for yourself and accomplish it and after you have celebrated your accomplishment, you need to set another goal for yourself. I realized that I was my own walking billboard and I had such a passion for sharing my knowledge. My good-living lifestyle was not something I wanted to keep secret. I wanted to share it with the world. So I started my own health coaching business. It was exciting and scary all at the same time but without taking a risk I wouldn't be where I am today. I am a successful entrepreneur and a proud business owner. Naturally, I continue to set new goals for myself and my ambition to learn more and more never stops.

Post IIN, I knew there was more to my own personal journey. I knew that I had to dig even deeper. You know the old saying "Ask and you shall receive", so I asked myself, "What next?" Well, I received my next message loud and clear. Through IIN, I was introduced to Holistic MBA where I earned my masters in TCM (transformational coaching methods).

Long story short, for the past thirty years I have chosen to live my happiest, healthiest life. My training/schooling has helped me reach my desires and goals of begin a rockin', healthy, happy, 50-year-old hockey mom of two teenagers.

I am blessed to have found my purpose, my calling. Through my life coaching business I help others find appreciation in their present state but then we look deeper and out into their future to uncover what it is that they now desire; what is it that they want three steps beyond their current state?

Let's get back to you and your desires to become the elite hockey player you desire to be. By taking the initiative to incorporate healthier eating habits and wrapping your mind around living a clean lifestyle and setting goals for yourself, who says you can't become a pro hockey player? I say, "Go for it!"

As a young athlete you might not even be thinking about such life-threatening diseases as those which my parents battled. In fact, I imagine the only thing that you can think about is playing hockey, but let me tell you, you will be so grateful you made these changes while you were an active athlete. There will be the day when you put your stick down. However, you won't have to end up as a couch potato, overweight, smoking, drinking and popping pills to combat an unhealthy lifestyle, because you learned what to avoid and how to eat the right foods NOW. How awesome is that?

You are AWESOME!

2

ON-THE-RUN/EATING OUT

Let's start with eating on-the-run and having to grab a meal here and there. Let's face it, you're a hockey player and there's not a whole lot of opportunity to eat at home because often your schedule has you at the rink during dinner hour or too early in the morning to even fix breakfast. Please don't put too much pressure on yourself, nor your parents, if the only choice you have is to grab something on the go and it is from a fast food joint. I know. I know. You may be just mortified that I'm saying that it's ok to eat out . . . like at a *McDonald's!?* It is—just give me a chance and I'll explain.

My kids and I catch a lot of flak when we are seen at a McDonald's drive-thru with our "HEALTHY" license plate on our car but I will never be embarrassed nor stressed out about eating at McDonald's because I know what to order to keep it healthy for me and my family and I look forward to sharing those healthy choices with you too. But please keep in mind that sometimes it's more than just about the meal. Sometimes it's about feeding your soul.

Over thirteen years ago I met one of my very best friends at a McDonald's. No lie! This friendship has been one of the most precious friendships of my life. If we hadn't gone to McDonald's on that frigid, winter Minnesota day back in February 2001, we wouldn't have met Karen and Benjamin. My son, Hayden, was just a little shy of two years old and my daughter, Leah, was *only* six weeks old.

None of us will ever forget that fateful day. Hayden was full of energy and I just had to get him someplace where he could simply tear around. My choice? McDonald's Play Place. I plunked myself down in a booth and, with Leah in her car-seat carrier, I placed her right on top of the table. Babies do attract people, that's for sure. And, as sure as a whirl, Karen struck up a conversation with me. She does this with every stranger. Karen has more friends than I've ever known a person to have. She's genuine. She wants to know all about you and she will care for you for the rest of your life.

Anyhoo, before our first visit was over, she was handing me a slip of paper which had her phone number on it. Naturally, I called the next day and left a message with Karen's husband, Bill. We get such a kick out of sharing the story of how Bill passed along the message. He said, "Karen, your McDonald's friend called." To this day that's how we refer to one another with introductions. Imagine being a health coach and being introduced to folks as "this is my McDonald's friend"! Too funny. Ben was my son's first true buddy and my daughter's very first friend. The three of them refer to each other as brother and sister. With so little family, we are forever grateful for the Healy family.

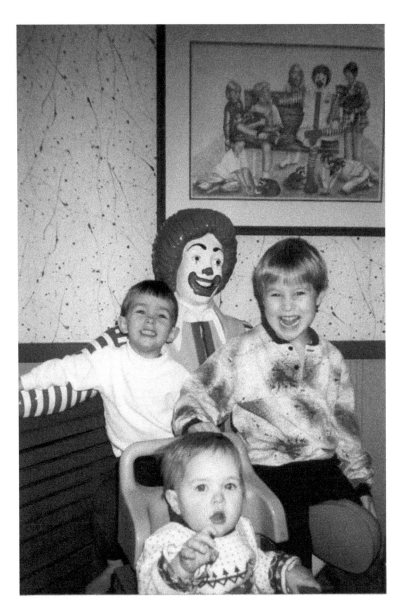

Hayden, Leah & Ben (January 2002)

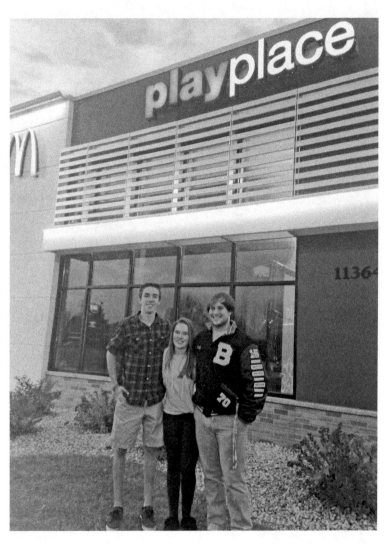

Hayden, Leah & Ben (October 2014)

Anyway, I'll bet you, yourself, once played at a McDonald's Play Place. In fact, I know you have if you were born and raised in Minnesota. It's almost a law, no, I'm not kidding you. Winters are so long and hard that parents would simply go out of their minds if they didn't have the McDonald's Play Place to escape to with their little ones to get them out of the house and get some place where they can wear their kids OUT! Either that or parents with toddlers would be drinking by noon from mid-November through March, or even into April. Wait! That sounds like our hockey season! Well, have you ever survived a Minnesota winter? Then, please don't judge. Minnesotans are beautiful and hardy people and they know how to enjoy their long winters.

In all seriousness, if the universe steers you to a fast food establishment, trust the vortex, *the pull*, because you never know who you just might meet. Always keep in mind that friendships are necessary for a happy and healthy life.

Never be embarrassed or stressed out over having to eat out when there is no other choice. We are *all* doing the best we can with what we know and what we have. So, that being said, if a fast food place is your only option, who cares? No one knows what you're getting while cruising through the drive-thru and, quite frankly, it's no one's business, now, is it?

Let me share with you some ideas when having to eat on-the-run, though please note that under the Recipes chapter I have provided you with healthier, homemade versions of some your favorite foods from such places as Chipotle.

Please keep in mind the one thing that worries me the most about eating out is the amount of sodium found in the foods you're eating. It is recommended that teenage boys, between the ages of 14 and 18, should consume no more than 1500 mg of sodium per day. On average you guys are consuming around 4500 mg per day! I am attempting to provide you with healthier choices which won't cause your ankles to swell and your face to completely break out with zits. (Please refer to the Chapter 3 for more information on sodium and its functions in the body.)

MCDONALD'S

McDonald's is the place to meet friends . . . okay, seriously, the grilled chicken snack wrap with no sauce is an okay choice. Grab one of the salads (Caution: by adding chicken you may end up with too much sodium) and skip the dressing. "A salad without dressing", you ask? Sure. Give it a try. It's a novel idea, I know, to actually taste the delicious vegetables beautifully thrown all together without needing to douse it with salad dressing. Ask for unsweetened, iced tea with lemon. Grab a fat-free/low-fat/skim milk. See, that's not so bad, is it? Here are a few other options:

- 1% low-fat, white or chocolate milk
- Apple slices
- Fruit and walnut salad
- Fruit and maple oatmeal
- Side salad (skip dressings, enjoy the taste)
- Hamburger
- Cheeseburger
- Grilled chicken sandwich (no sauce)
- Grilled chicken snack wrap (no sauce/lower in sodium)
- Egg McMuffin®
- Scrambled eggs (lower in sodium)
- Unsweetened iced tea (with or without lemon)

Yes, in this case at McDonald's the hamburger and cheese-burger have less sodium than sandwiches/wraps made with grilled chicken. So, if your body is craving a hamburger, get one. I even tell my vegetarian clients that if they are craving a burger, eat a burger. I tell them to pay attention to what their body is craving. Cravings are a sure sign that your body is missing some kind of nutrient that is missing. If you're craving red meat you may be low on iron. Just opt for a regular burger or cheeseburger, a no frills burger.

JIMMY JOHN'S

Jimmy John's can be a place to run to if you are needing to bulk up, to build muscle, by grabbing a regular sandwich; the combination of proteins and carbs will help add some "meat to your bones." However, again, I caution you regarding having a sandwich because just one alone has you close to your daily recommended sodium intake; stick with the turkey. As you can gather, I, personally, am not a big fan of bread. So what shall you consider if Jimmy John's is the chosen spot to eat? Have you ever tried Jimmy John's "unwich"? Here's a time to try something new. Once, I offered my son's friend, Cole, to try an unwich on me and if he didn't care for it after two bites (that's my rule) he didn't have to eat it. Post meal, Cole asked if he could move in with us. You will find the unwich to be the most marvelous sandwich you will ever have that doesn't come with bread, it is wrapped up beautifully in lettuce. It can be a little tricky when eating your first unwich. Unwrap bit-by-bit, otherwise it can come apart and that will just frustrate you. WARNING: The unwich will become your new addiction.

- Unwich
- Water
- Unsweetened iced tea

SUBWAY

Subways are everywhere and can be a convenient spot to replenish post game or in-between games. I am going to suggest you try their chopped salad and have them add a scoop of the tuna for a little added protein. Have them add the banana peppers, jalapeño peppers and olives for a nice punch of flavor then you won't need any salad dressing. Remember now, that the meats can carry a lot of sodium.

- Chopped Salad
- Apple Slices
- Water

CHIPOTLE

I believe Chipotle may be the new favorite amongst teenagers. Burritos with meat/chicken, beans, rice, veggies, salsa, sour cream and guacamole—it all sounds good, doesn't it? No! It's horrific! Hideous! How many of your friends look like they've packed on the old "freshmen 15" . . . not familiar with that term? Ask your parents. You have got to stay educated and share your knowledge with others. Please look up the nutritional facts and you'll throw up. The amount of sodium is off-the-hook! Not to mention the unhealthy amounts of fat and unwanted calories. Yes, as a hockey player, you burn a lot of calories but if dining on this kind of food becomes a habit, it will become a very bad habit and you'll be sorry.

But, if this is where everyone is going between tournament games, here are the only choices I would recommend for you:

- Soft, corn tortilla with brown rice, black beans & cheese
- Burrito bowl, with brown rice, black beans & cheese

- Salad, with romaine, brown rice, black beans & cheese

Sorry if I'm scaring you. Well, no I'm not sorry but I have good news. I have my homemade Mexican food alternative under the Recipe chapter for you to make yourself and enjoy without endangering your body.

Okay, so those are about the only places I'm going to suggest because really, deep down, I want you to avoid eating out as much as you can and begin to embrace the importance of attempting to prepare your meals at home whenever possible. But don't stress out if you're grabbing on-the-go, sometimes there's no choice.

Moving on to the good stuff . . .

3

PROTEIN, CARBS, FATS & SODIUM

Having fun yet? I sure hope you're learning a lot and that you're really beginning to think twice about what you're putting into your body and, just think, we've only just begun. No, the fun doesn't stop here. :) I am a total advocate of having fun and being relaxed. I ask you to please celebrate the investment you've made to become knowledgeable in understanding what is right for YOU. I can't express this enough, we are all bio-individuals and there is no one diet or formula to teach. I will give you guidelines but it's up to you (*the puck stops here*) to pay attention. Better yet, journal about it. Remember, start keeping track of how you feel when you eat certain foods and when you drink certain beverages. How much was too much and/or how much was not enough? Did you have more energy or less? How was your concentration? Did your stomach settle nicely or did you get a gut bomb? You will find the perfect formula for you by experimenting with it and making note of it.

PROTEIN

Lean protein is important to have at each meal. It builds tissue, repairs cells, balances blood sugar and body fluids. Protein helps to build up your immune system. It increases your metabolism and it makes hormones and enzymes, all of which are important in order for your body to function at its best. If you want to sport an awesome "flow" with thick, healthy hair and strong nails to dig into your opponent (just kidding) and fabulous, zit-free skin, be sure to get enough protein.

Okay, as for protein, the daily recommendation is:

Girls (14-18 years old):   46 grams
Boys (14-18 years old):   52 grams
Women (ages 19-70+):   46 grams
Men (ages 19-70+):   56 grams

However, for elite athletes such as yourself, it has been recommended that you should consume between .5-.8 grams of protein per pound. Example: A 200-lb hockey player should eat 100-160 grams of protein per day. Here's the math: 200 x .5 = 100 as minimum or 200 x .8 = 160 as the maximum.

In the next chapter you will find a list of recommended lean proteins.

CARBS

There are two kinds of carbohydrates, simple and complex.

Simple carbohydrates are easily and rapidly digested and are the quickest source of energy. Simple carbohydrates food sources:

- Fruits
- Vegetables
- Table sugar
- Brown sugar
- Honey
- Maple syrup
- Molasses
- Jams, jellies

Here are some more, but I want you to stay away from these in particular:

- Fruit drinks
- Soft drinks
- Candy
- Corn syrup

Complex carbohydrates are sometimes referred to as a starch. They are high in <u>fiber</u>. They help make you feel satiated (full) and they can help promote good health.

Complex carbs are found in whole plant foods and can be high in minerals and vitamins. Sources of complex carbs:

- Green vegetables
- Oatmeal
- Pasta
- Whole-grain breads
- Potatoes
- Sweet potatoes
- Corn
- Pumpkin
- Beans

- Lentils
- Peas

You get your primary source of energy from carbohydrates. How many carbohydrates should one consume on game days? Hockey players (elite athletes) need carbohydrates for performance and endurance on the ice.

Here's the math: A 190 lb. player x 4.5g = 855g of carbohydrates; 1g carb = 4 cals; 855g x 4c = 3420 carb calories.

FATS

Incorporating healthy fats into your daily diet is imperative for absorbing vitamins, optimizing digestion and for your cognitive function. What does cognitive function mean? It has everything to do with your decision making, your problem solving, adding, subtracting, multiplying, dividing—you know, all of that mathematic stuff, plus, speaking and memory, the ability to remember lots of important things. In the next chapter you will find a list of recommended healthy fats.

SODIUM

I realize I have been preaching heavily to you about the importance of not consuming too much salt but your body does need sodium in order to function properly. Sodium helps your body maintain its fluid levels; your body must have sodium to work together with important minerals such as potassium and calcium (also known as electrolytes) to keep things in balance. Sodium is essential to help control your blood pressure and blood volume. It also ensures that your nerves and muscles are working properly.

It's time to take out your journal again and keep note of how much sodium you're consuming in a day because too much sodium can be deadly over periods of time. Do your parents or grandparents have high blood pressure? Do you know of anyone who has had a heart attack? Over time, if you consume excessive amounts of sodium, you, too, will likely end up with heart issues, with life-threatening problems such as a heart attack or cardiovascular disease.

On average, healthy adults should *only* consume between 1500 mg to 2300 mg of sodium per day and, again, for the average teenager around 1500 mg per day. FYI, 1 teaspoon of table salt contains around 2300 mg of sodium. Simply pay attention to the amount of sodium per serving on nutrition labels. If one morning you wake up and you feel all "puffy," more than likely there was a tremendous amount of added salt in the meals you consumed the day before.

The easiest lesson for me to teach you is to recommend that you taste your meal prior to picking up the salt shaker. You will probably find your meal salty enough without adding more salt. More than likely, there was enough salt added during preparation and, remember, adding more salt can be deadly. Be aware that most foods naturally contain sodium.

Food naturally containing sodium:

- Table salt
- Milk
- Beets
- Celery

Watch for added sodium in:

- Processed meats
- Bacon
- Sausage
- Ham
- Canned soups and vegetables
- Worcestershire sauce
- Soy sauce
- Onion salt
- Garlic salt
- Bouillon cubes

Sodium can be listed on labels under these names:

- monosodium glutamate
- sodium nitrite
- sodium saccharin
- baking soda (sodium bicarbonate)

Too much sodium in the diet may lead to:

- High blood pressure
- Congestive heart failure
- Cirrhosis of the liver
- Kidney disease

4

FUELING & REFUELING
FOR GAMES/PRACTICES

TIMING

The most common question is when to eat *before* and *after* games and practices.

Pre-Game/Practice:

To best prepare your body for your highest level of performance, p*re-game or practice,* it is recommended that you eat two hours or ninety minutes prior to and to drink 16-20 oz. of water. Pay attention to which worked better for you: two hours before or ninety minutes before your game/practice. Write down your results in your food journal. Tweak the timing depending on how you felt during your game/practice. How was your energy level? Did you play incredibly strong for all three periods? Did your energy level begin to wane after the second period or even after the first? Did you feel like you had a "gut bomb." In other words, did your stomach feel heavy and sluggish? How was your concentration level? Were you able to focus throughout the entire game? If not, when did you start to lose focus? If you aren't able to write it down, certainly make a mental note of it. This is the only way you'll find the best answers for you.

Easy-to-grab meal pre-game/practice:

To get instant energy, drink a tall glass of milk and eat some fruit. This is great in the mornings because it's an easily digestible meal. It's important to eat an easily digestible meal in the mornings because between the hours of 6:00 a.m. and noon your body is using energy to digest the foods you ate the night before.

Post-Game/Practice:

If possible, try to eat within 45 minutes after your game or practice, the following will explain why.

Easy-to-grab meal for post-game/practice:

For muscle recovery dine on an apple and 1-2 oz. of nuts, and enjoy with a bottle of water.

HYDRATING

I recommended that you are drinking pure, filtered water and that you're drinking at least half of your body weight in ounces per day, every day. More is recommended on your game days. So for example, if you weigh 120 pounds you need to drink 60 ounces of water.

To help promote the energy that you need during your game/practice drink 4-6 oz. of water every 15 minutes.

Post game/practice you'll need to drink lots and lots of water. For every pound you lose post game/practice you will need to consume 16 oz. of water to replace it.

Water is essential to transport nutrients throughout your body, and your immune system relies on fluids to flush out toxins. This helps keep colds and flu at bay.

Could you be dehydrated? If you are feeling tired and sluggish, dehydration is more than likely the culprit. Are you feeling parched? Another clear indication of dehydration is when one is feeling parched. When you go to the bathroom, what color is your pee? If it's dark yellow you are not getting enough water. Drinking warm water is more hydrating than cold water. So enjoy hot tea or soups as another way to increase your fluids.

When traveling by airplane to your tournaments be sure to properly hydrate your body. For every hour you are on the plane drink 20 oz. of water.

Want to jazz things up a bit with your water intake and improve your energy level? Add some sliced fruit to your water to give it a little flavor. Or, if you're a fan, drink coconut water. If you're not too keen on the flavor of coconut itself there are many brands out there which offer other flavors such as chocolate, mango, pineapple and pink guava. Try my green lemonade* recipe under the Recipe chapter. Kombucha is a nice thing to grab and it's naturally fizzy, kind of like drinking a soda but healthy for you.

CARBOHYDRATES

When it comes to understanding how many carbohydrates you should consume on game day, again, that will depend upon finding the best balance for you. Approximately 60% of what is on your plate should be complex carbohydrates. If you picture your plate, that would be a little more than half of your plate. Complex carbohydrates help you sustain energy for peak performance and provide fuel for your muscles.

Great sources of carbs:

- Bouncing Biscuits™ (recipe included)
- Green Dream Smoothie™ (recipe included)
- Fruit and/or veggie smoothie
- Baked potato, sweet potato
- Pasta
- Brown rice (not white rice, it has zero nutrients)
- Beans
- Banana (simple carb/simple sugar, great energy)
- Oatmeal (add Skoop™, nuts and/or fruit)
- Ezekiel bread with almond butter or natural peanut butter with banana slices
- Fruits—bananas, in particular
- Vegetables
- Quinoa
- Vegetable soup
- Rice crackers
- Pretzels

Crappy carbs to AVOID: Soda, candy, desserts, white bread, baked treats, bagels, coffee with sugar and syrups, ice cream and anything made with white sugar or bleached flour.

After games it's important to replenish your energy levels by creating a meal which consists of 50% good complex carbohydrates.

LEAN PROTEIN

Along with your carbs you want to add lean protein to your meal, both before and after games/practices. Lean proteins should take up about 30% of your plate. Looking at your plate now, there's only a sliver left uncovered. That last 10% is designated for healthy fats. Lean protein before a game helps prevent muscle breakdown and aids in muscle recovery post-game. The beauty of protein is that it makes you feel full, balances your blood sugar and body fluids, and it helps to repair and build the cells in your body. Lean protein helps to build up your immune system so that you don't miss practices or games because of colds and/or the flu. Lean protein increases your metabolism and makes essential hormones and enzymes, all which your body needs to keep it healthy and balanced.

The best place to pick up lean meat is from your local butcher shop or at the butcher counter of your local grocery store. You can hand-select what you want and have it packaged fresh right then and there.

Great sources of lean protein (not just meat):

- Steak
- Fish
- Bison
- Ostrich
- Turkey

- Chicken
- Organic, Greek yogurt with fruit and B-Strong Skoop™
- Eggs, egg whites
- Cheese
- Cottage cheese
- Fat-free/low-fat/skim milk
- Beans, legumes
- Quinoa

Remember, lean protein post games/practices help to build upon your existing muscles and help rebuild torn down muscles.

HEALTHY FATS

It is important to add a little bit of healthy fats to your meal, about 10% to 20% pre- and post-games/practices.

The benefits of having small amounts of healthy fats:

- Balances blood sugar
- Helps the body utilize vitamins A, D, E and K
- Slows down digestion
- Great for concentration

Great sources of healthy oils:

- Olive oil
- Coconut oil
- Avocados
- Nuts

5

PACKING A COOLER

A couple of years ago, between games of a grueling tournament, everyone was asking, "What should we be feeding our
kids before the next game?!"

It was then that I realized I needed to share with the coaches
that I was a health coach. At that time, my health coaching
practice had mainly consisted of women ages 30 to 70 but all
of a sudden I realized that here was a group of teens needing
some nutritional training—parents, too, for those that were
interested. I mentioned to the coaches that I would be de-
lighted to work with the team to help them get educated and
embrace the importance of not only on- and off-ice training
but what was going into the bodies of these young, growing
athletes.

The coaches loved the idea and so began my health-coaching
for hockey players. Between tournament games I educated
the players on proper nutrition (I still offer group programs
should you be interested for you and your team). I started
to bring along my Vitamix to all of the tournaments; it even

had its own suitcase. The players used to line up in the hotel hallway or meet me in the hotel lobby waiting for my return from Costco with fruits, veggies and Greek yogurt. Together the players and I would whip up smoothies and each and every time they would out-perform their opponents in terms of energy and endurance.

Many of my clients asked that I create a "cooler plan" so that they are always prepared and needn't grab fast food on-the-go. I designed the cooler plan for the growing athlete and for the athlete who needs to eat five to six meals throughout the day.

I recommend you fill your cooler with lean proteins, complex carbohydrates and healthy beverages that are low in sugar and low in sodium.

Easy-to-grab meal pre-game/practice:

A bottle of water along with a sandwich made on whole wheat bread with lean turkey breast (fresh, not processed), cheese, lettuce and tomato with a dab of mayo or mustard.

LEAN PROTEINS/CARBS
- grilled, baked or broiled chicken/turkey (size of a deck-of-cards or your palm; 2-5 x per day)
- tuna or salmon (1 package in water, if desired, mix with mayo; 1 x per day, not every day, though)
- grilled, baked, broiled or poached fish (white fish or salmon)
- hard-boiled eggs (1-2 per meal, once or twice per day)

- cottage cheese or cheese sticks (1 cup per day/2-4 per day)
- Greek yogurt (1-2 cups per day)
- kefir (1-2 cups per day)
- raw, unsalted nuts (1 handful per day)
- sunflower seeds (1 handful per day)
- pumpkin seeds (1 handful per day)
- natural peanut butter (2-4 tablespoons per day)
- almond butter (2-4 tablespoons per day)
- apples (2 small per day)
- pears (1 per day)
- oranges/tangerines/clementines (2 small per day)
- berries (1/2 cup 2-4 x per day)
- melon (1/2 cup 2-4 x per day)
- banana (1 per day)
- cucumbers/zucchini (1 cup per day)
- celery (1-3 stalks per day)
- carrots (1/2-1 cup per day)
- tomatoes (1 cup per day)
- broccoli (1 cup per day)
- asparagus (1 cup per day)
- green beans (1 cup per day)
- peppers (red, yellow, orange, green; 1 cup per day)
- vegetable soup (1 Thermos full per day)
- bell peppers (1 cup per day)
- cooked sweet potato or baked potato (1 per day)
- whole-grain bread or wraps (1-2 slices per day)
- cooked quinoa, brown rice or oatmeal* (1-2 cups per day)

*For more energy add 2 tablespoons of ground flaxseed and/or chia seeds or a scoop of B-Strong protein powder available at http://coachloves.healthyskoop.com)

BEVERAGES

- water/coconut waters
- smoothie*
- herbal, decaf tea
- homemade energy drinks
- V8 Fusion
- low-sodium V8
- almond milk
- skim/fat-free or 1% milk (FairLife™ is higher in protein, less sugar than other brands)
- Aspire™ energy drinks

*For more energy add a scoop of A-Game powder available at http://coachloves.healthyskoop.com)

TIP FOR PARENTS AT TOURNAMENTS (WINK! WINK!):

One of the quickest ways of curing a hangover is to have a glass of milk and a banana. The banana will help calm your stomach and assist with regulating your blood sugar levels and the milk with help re-hydrate and soothe your system. It neutralizes an over-acidic stomach.

6

TIPS FOR ENDURANCE & ENERGY

In this section I am going to provide you with a few tips/suggestions on ways to help your body preserve and/or create energy. Thus, your endurance levels will improve while out on the ice during practices and games.

GOOD OL' WATER

Yes, naturally, I am going to repeat myself over and over again and tell you to *drink water*! I know, I know, but it is critical that this healthy habit just becomes second nature. Though, don't go super crazy with the amount of water you drink. Drinking too much water can be deadly. How much should you drink again? The rule-of-thumb is half your body weight in ounces, more on game days. Avoid any beverages with caffeine, such as soda pop, it will dehydrate you and it will cause your blood sugar to go up and down.

HEALTHY BALANCE OF ANIMAL PROTEIN

Be aware that by eating too much animal protein (red meat, chicken, eggs and dairy) can actually rob you of good energy levels. However, a lack of enough animal protein can also be an issue. Pay attention to your body—what is it craving? How is your energy level? Which lean animal protein helped and which wreaked havoc on your energy level? Again, keep track in your journal exactly which proteins seemed to bring you the most energy.

DARK, LEAFY GREENS

Throughout the hockey season indulge in dark, leafy greens but don't stop post-season because, as spring time approaches, be aware that it is your body's time for renewal. DLGs (dark, leafy greens) are refreshing and will provide you with the vital energy you are wanting, plus, they are chockfull of vitamins and nutrients, all of which improve your circulation. And *that* is a great tip to share with your parents! If your folks are complaining about being too cold in the rink, suggest they eat more DLGs. It helps get their blood moving and they'll feel warm all over. DLGs purify your blood and strengthen your immune system; what better way to prevent you from getting a cold or the flu? So plan on eating lots of things like kale, arugula, broccoli, collards, bok choy, mustard greens, broccoli rabe, beet and dandelion greens.

QUINOA

Quinoa has as much protein as a glass of milk and is considered a complete protein because it contains all eight amino acids. It is high in B vitamins, iron, zinc, potassium, calcium, and vitamin E. Plus, quinoa is gluten-free and easy to digest.

Therefore, quinoa is the ideal food for endurance, plus, it strengthens your kidneys, heart, and lungs. So, if you would like to switch it up a bit, have some quinoa instead of oatmeal.

NATURALLY SWEET TREATS

Prior to your game or in-between games or periods, reach for naturally sweet treats such as a banana, pear, apple or an orange along with a tall glass of milk. Please do not reach for sugary foods such as donuts or pastries to get a short-lived energy boost. It is important to try to avoid sugar and, in particular, any artificial sweeteners.

COCONUT OIL

Did you know that coconut oil can boost your thyroid function, resulting in an increase in metabolism, energy and endurance? Yep, it's that simple. The next time you sauté vegetables, sauté using coconut oil in lieu of olive oil.

By now, I hope, you are beginning to really embrace the fact that it is critical for you to eat well and stay hydrated to increase your energy and endurance levels. But how about considering a few more things, things such as:

ADEQUATE SLEEP

Are you getting enough sleep? The optimal number of hours of sleep to get in a night is 7.5 to 8 hours but a growing teenage athlete will likely need more. Get to bed early the night before games. Turn off your smartphone, the TV, X-Box/Playstation and grab a book to help relax your brain. A tired and stressed out body completely deprives your body of any energy. When you are sleep-deprived due to going to bed late and waking up early, you will crave unhealthy things such as sugar and caffeine and those would be horrible to have prior to your game. Right? You betcha!

DIGESTION

As I mentioned before, keep in mind that your body is busy digesting and processing the foods you ate the night before. Your liver begins its detox function around 3:00 a.m. and your digestive system kicks into gear around 6:00 a.m. and is busy at work until around noon. Can you just imagine how much energy your body is expending digesting the foods from the night before? Pasta is a good choice the night before a game but don't overload in the morning with a heavy breakfast. Grab something like a bowl of oatmeal with fruit and enjoy it with a tall glass of milk.

MEDITATE

Get in touch with your spiritual side. Meditate, dance, go to church/temple or step out into nature and take the time to appreciate your beautiful surroundings. Taking advantage of opportunities to tap into your spiritual being will make you feel like a million bucks. You will experience an incredible energy boost.

HAVE A LITTLE FUN

I know it's hard to find the time to do other activities you enjoy when you're on the ice six days a week or, in some cases, fourteen days straight; but you can restore your energy by taking time for yourself. Go to the movies, play a board game, read a book, listen to your favorite music, hang out with friends and family—whatever it is that you enjoy, DO IT! A change of pace and scene will rejuvenate you.

BEAUTIFUL GARDEN OF FRIENDS

Any chance you have any relationships/friendships that just drain you? Too much drama? Folks can drain you of your energy, particularly if there's a lot of drama involved. Those individuals aren't bad, but it is important to pay attention to who tends to drain you and why. A dear friend (thank you, Ellen) of mine once helped explain this to me by having me picture my life and its surroundings like a beautiful garden. Sometimes there are "weeds" amongst the beauty. We need not kill off the "weeds" but we can "fence" them off from the rest of our beautiful garden.

Set boundaries with those individuals who drain you of your energy levels, or attempt to transform the relationship with open and honest communication. As I learned from my mentors (thank you Carey and Stacey), please understand that all acts are either an act of love or a cry for love.

In my next book, I will go into greater detail about relationships. In the meantime, I ask that you keep in mind that our loved ones are always doing the best that they can with what they have and what they know. Your loved ones' actions are never intended to be hurtful.

7

THINGS TO AVOID—GET TOTALLY GROSSED OUT!

Right off the bat, here are just few things to avoid; memorize this list:

- Saturated fats
- Trans fats
- Processed foods like deli meat and cheeses
- Preservatives
- Refined flour
- Sugar
- Zero-nutrient foods and beverages

STEROIDS!

Were you aware that steroids have been associated with shrunken testicles and breast enlargement in males; sounds like a real problem, doesn't it? Growth hormone and anabolic steroids can cause such issues. Plus, they can screw up your metabolism. Steroids can cause tumors and destroy joints. Not to mention the possibility of getting HIV, hepatitis or other infections by using shared needles to inject steroids. Do you think your hockey idol ever used steroids? Heavens no! They built their bodies the old-fashioned way by eating real whole foods and pumping iron.

SODA POP! *STOP* DRINKING IT!

Here is something totally gross! Are you aware of the amount of sugar in a 16 oz. bottle of regular soda? There are 10 tsp. of sugar in one bottle! Picture 15 cubes of sugar crammed into one bottle. That's no lie. Not to mention the wasteful 100-200 empty calories.

Please, never drink another soda pop again! I'll give you a couple of reasons why . . .

#1 Soda Pop Causes Dehydration

Soda pop does not quench your thirst. In fact, it is loaded with caffeine and it acts like a diuretic, causing you to pee more often, thus, leaving you dehydrated. It's never good when you need to leave the rink to go to the bathroom during a game; now is it?

#2 Soda Pop Can Cause Lower Bone Density

Want your bones to easily break when getting checked into the boards? Go ahead and drink soda pop. Back in the "old days," around the 1950s, studies show that kids used to consume three cups of milk a day. Today, kids are drinking three glasses of pop. Soda pop should not be your replacement drink. Please, please, please pick healthier options. More and more folks are struggling with low-bone density. Thus we're seeing more and more cases of osteoporosis in children, women and men; you don't want to be an adult who's all hunched over—not pretty.

#3 Soda Pop is Said to Deplete Minerals

My son once did a science project in which he soaked chicken bones in three separate containers. One container had cola, one had milk and the other water. After two weeks he removed the bones from their containers. The bone soaked in cola was nasty in color and when he bent the bone it snapped easily in half. The one soaked in water remained the same color and wasn't as easy to snap in half, yet the one soaked in milk was bright white and was the hardest to break in half. Most colas contain phosphoric acid and caffeine, both of which are said to remove calcium from your bones. And, since caffeine acts as a diuretic and increases the need to go to the bathroom, more minerals are exiting your body before they have a chance to be absorbed.

#4 Soda Pop is High in Acid

A body high in acid is inviting over 150 possible diseases including cancer, diabetes, gall and kidney stones, heart disease and arthritis, to name a few. That should scare you enough right now to quit drinking it. No? You want more . . . ok . . . So your body's optimal pH level is between 7 – 7.5 pH. The lower the pH number, i.e. 0, the more acidic, whereas 14 is totally alkaline. Again, you want to be right in the middle. When you drink soda (doesn't matter whether it's diet or regular), over time the acid in soda breaks down the enamel in your teeth and they can become weak, super sensitive and more susceptible to decay; hockey can already be hazardous to your pearly whites . . . why add risk to your gorgeous teeth by drinking soda pop? Here's something crazy! In tests done on the acidity levels of pop, pop was found to have a pH of 2.5. To help put that into perspective, the acid in a battery has a pH of 1, whereas pure water has a pH level of 7. Holy Hannah!

#5 Soda Pop is High in Sugar and Wasteful Calories

Look at the label on your soda bottle or can. One can of cola contains 100 to 200 calories and 10 teaspoons of sugar. An adult should consume no more than 10 teaspoons of added sugar in a day. That means one can of pop could meet the daily requirement of added sugar; please share that with your friends and family. Basically, ZERO nutritional value in soda, folks.

#6 Again, Caffeine in Soda Pop

Plain and simple, caffeine can be addictive. A study at Johns Hopkins University revealed a few interesting facts about caffeine. "Caffeine is the world's most commonly used stimulant, and it's cheap and readily available so people can maintain their use of caffeine quite easily," says Roland Griffiths, Ph.D., professor of psychiatry and neuroscience at Johns Hopkins. "The latest research demonstrates, however, that when people don't get their usual dose they can suffer a range of withdrawal symptoms, including headache, fatigue, and difficulty concentrating. They may even feel like they have the flu with nausea and muscle pain." So keep that in mind if you're feeling sick. It could just be the amount of soda your drinking.

#7 Artificial Sweeteners in Soda Pop

Drinking pop with artificial sweeteners can cause you to crave even more sweets. Evidently, there has been over 20 years of research behind artificial sweeteners, proving they are safe for most individuals. However, I do my best to steer my own kids away from beverages with artificial sweeteners.

#8 Avoid Getting Diabetes by Avoiding Soda Pop

While no research has definitively shown that pop causes diabetes, pop can bring on unwanted weight gain. According to a researcher from Children's Hospital Boston, the fact remains, "When sugar enters the bloodstream quickly, the pancreas has to secrete large amounts of insulin for the body to process it. Some scientists believe that the unceasing demands that a soda habit places on the pancreas may ultimately leave it unable to keep up with the body's need for insulin. Also, insulin itself becomes less effective at processing sugar; both conditions contribute to the risk of developing diabetes." Enough said.

#9 Do You Know Someone Who Wants to Lose Weight?

The word "diet" on a label is misleading and quite evil really. Researchers at the University of Texas Health Science Center found that *diet* sodas put a person at a higher risk of becoming overweight. According to their research, "Artificial sweeteners can interfere with the body's natural ability to regulate calorie intake. This could mean people who consume artificially-sweetened items are more likely to overindulge."

#10 Stop Buying Pop; It'll Save You Money

Soda may be considered inexpensive when compared to making your own homemade smoothie filled with high-in-nutrient fruits and vegetables. However, consider this: depending upon where you live, the price of a bottle of soda pop can average anywhere between $1 to $2. If you drank two a day at $2 per pop, you would be spending over $1400 on soda alone. Think how many hockey sticks you could buy. If you quit spending money on this useless beverage, you could buy yourself *top of the line* hockey skates. Share this savings with your parents; they could apply this money toward your ice-time invoice or toward the expenses of some of your tournaments.

Okay, enough about soda pop and why to avoid it, let's move on to another evil . . .

SUGAR—IT'S THE DEVIL!

There is ZERO nutritional value in the additive, sugar. It's only added to processed foods to make it taste better and get you craving more of the bad foods you think you are enjoying. Are you aware of the seriousness of avoiding sugar? It can cause serious short- and long-term health problems—things like excess weight gain, hormone imbalance, insulin resistance, skin issues, dental issues, osteoporosis, diabetes/obesity. It wreaks havoc on the immune system and it can possibly cause some forms of cancer, inflammatory diseases, fatigue and irritability. Sugar doesn't sound so good anymore, does it? Good!

What makes you crave sugar? Sugar cravings are caused by hormonal imbalance of estrogen and progesterone and insulin levels. When you consume too much sugar your hormones get all out of whack. Do you ever feel irritable, anxious or totally fatigued? Well, that's a sure sign that your testosterone, progesterone and estrogen levels are all out of balance and hormonal issues can lead to serious illnesses.

Have you ever craved sugar after a stressful event? Well, stress provokes cortisol to be released in your system and with increased cortisol levels you will have the urge to refuel on sugary foods/drinks. Thus, try to avoid all refined carbohydrates, also known as "comfort foods" after a stressful event.

How is the dreaded sugar roller coaster? Are you familiar with that? When you eat sugar your blood sugar and serotonin levels rise, endorphins kick in and you enter a place of euphoria. Your body reaches an amazing peak only to have your blood sugar suddenly plummet, just like being on a roller coaster. When this happens you lose concentration and you can get really cranky and all fatigued and your craving for sugar starts all over again. It's not a day at the amusement park, is it?

When consuming sugar (such as in soda pop) there's the awful possibility, make that a probability, of unwanted weight gain. When you consume too much sugar and your body doesn't burn it all up through activity, it becomes glycogen, which your liver, sadly, has to store. The liver then gets all clogged up and your body begins to create fat all throughout your body. As a result you end up with unwanted weight gain. Do you want to sport that lovely old "tire" around your mid-section or end up with "love handles" on your hips? Didn't think so.

I hope this makes you really think twice about eating foods high in sugar. Read the labels on the foods you're thinking about eating. If there is more than 5-10 grams of added sugar per serving listed on the nutrition label, put it back on the shelf. If you're needing an energy boost, sugar is not the answer. I suggest you strap on your skates, clear the ice on the pond, and get out there and play, play hard!

Even though I will continue to beg you to please reduce your sugar intake, don't get all stressed out at special family occasions. Enjoy the cake and ice cream when celebrating with family and friends but be mindful of portion size. Ask for just a sliver of cake and only one scoop of ice cream. On other occasions, skip the dessert altogether. Trust me, down the road you will be glad you did.

If you want to avoid getting sick and missing any of your games it is time you take responsibility for your immune system. You know the drill by now, sugar and processed foods tear up your immune system. Give your body what it is asking for. It's begging for you to nourish it with water and nutrient-dense foods, not sugary, empty-calorie foods and beverages. If you make smart choices and nourish your body with all of the essential vitamins and nutrients it craves, you'll find yourself staying healthy all year long, not just during your hockey season.

Sugar calculation? Teenagers should not have more than 20 to 32 grams (that's only 5-8 teaspoons) of added sugar per day. Rule of thumb, again, is ten or less grams of added sugar per serving. One cube of sugar is equal to four grams of sugar. Go to your pantry and pull out a box of cereal. Take a look at the nutritional value column: how many grams of sugar do you find? Now divide that number by four. That is the amount of sugar cubes for just one serving. YIKES! Disgusting, right? So, you can see that the number of sugar cubes/grams of sugar can add up quickly.

SUGAR CHALLENGE:

Let me propose a challenge. Try to refrain from eating foods with added sugar for three days. In three short days your serotonin and endorphin levels will balance out and wonderful things will begin to take place in your brain.

Here are a few things I suggest you do to be successful with this challenge:

1. Stick to one-ingredient foods, avoiding anything and everything that comes in a package.
2. Avoid all sport/energy drinks, soda and juice.
3. Drink water with sliced fruit or herbal teas (hot or over ice).

Good luck!

Take note in your journal about how you're feeling throughout the three days. Did you begin to experience a sense of calmness wash over you? Were you less irritable? Less cranky? Less moody? Did your energy levels return or seem to improve?

After the three, short days the neurotransmitters in your brain will no longer send out signals asking for more sugar, You will have begun the process of no longer craving sugary foods. Pretty amazing, huh? Let me know how you did; send me an email at NHLhealthcoach@gmail.com.

SYNTHETIC VITAMINS

Synthetic vitamins are not easily absorbed by the body. When you take a synthetic vitamin often a lot of the vitamin's benefit exits your precious body when you take a pee. The best way to have all the necessary nutrients and phytonutrients absorbed by your body is by eating superfoods.

MEAT AND REFINED CARBS

Meat and refined carbs cause inflammation in the body. Eating a lot of meat and refined carbs tends to increase inflammation and acidity, causing the body to crave sweet foods. Anti-inflammatory foods high in omega-3 fatty acids, which are alkalizing and antioxidant-rich, such as fruits and veggies, can offset the damage and the cravings associated with this dynamic.

STRESS

Stressful situations can lead to poor eating habits. *Stress* increases cortisol levels, which increases hunger and one might experience nighttime cravings and over-eating. Over time, one can be faced with adrenal imbalance and extreme exhaustion. Thus, one will drink lots of caffeine and consume sugar for quick energy bursts. Avoid both. Exercise instead.

GMOs

Genetically Modified Organisms are plants/animals which have been created through gene splicing techniques or, in other terms, genetically engineered "GE". DNA is merged together from different species, creating unstable combinations of plant, animal, bacterial and viral genes which does not occur in nature or in traditional crossbreeding.

There are more and more studies pointing to human health risks with GMOs. There is a cause for concern with regards to food allergies, irritable bowel syndrome, organ damage and even cancer.

Here are some of the most common GMOs:

- Alfalfa
- Canola
- Corn
- Cotton
- Soy

ALSO high-risk because of contamination in feed:

- Animal products
- Milk
- Meat
- Eggs
- Honey

How can you further avoid GMOs? Eat out less often and when buying groceries:

- Look for the non-GMO Project label, be wary of non-GMO claims that lack certification
- Buy organic certified produce and packaged foods
- Avoid processed foods

PRESERVATIVES TO AVOID

Moving on to more things which are added to processed foods which can be harmful to your health. The list is really quite endless but I'm giving you the really good stuff. This has been interesting, hasn't it?

Preservative—BHA

BHA (butylated hydroxyanisole) . . . can't pronounce it? Nor can I. My rule of thumb . . . if you can't pronounce it don't put it in your mouth. Anyway, BHA is used to help foods which contain oils from becoming rancid. BHA has been shown to cause cancer in lab rats and mice. The cancers all occurred in the *fore stomachs* of the rodents, the fore stomach is an organ that we humans don't have; hence, FDA has not banned it from being used. Nevertheless, the study, published in the *Japanese Journal of Cancer Research*, concluded that BHA was "reasonably anticipated to be a carcinogen." That's reason enough to eliminate it from your diet; wouldn't you agree?

Food(s) which may have BHA: sugary cereals

Preservative—Paraben

To inhibit mold and yeast in food the synthetic preservative paraben is used. The problem is paraben may disrupt your body's hormones. If ingested daily, a study in *Food Chemical Toxicology* found decreased sperm and testosterone production in rats. Breast cancer tissues have also shown signs of paraben in them.

Food(s) which may have paraben: ice cream

Partially Hydrogenated Oil

Partially hydrogenated oil is an artery-clogging trans fat. Please don't confuse "zero trans fat" with being trans fat-*free*. The FDA allows companies to claim "zero grams of trans fat" if it contains less than half a gram per serving. No more than two grams is what an individual should consume in a day.

But even 1/2 of a gram can add up quickly and if it's listed as "zero" then you may not be aware that you're even having a 1/2 of a gram; those fractions can quickly add up. Watch for partially hydrogenated oil on ingredient labels; if it's anywhere on label try to skip the item altogether.

Food(s) which may have partially hydrogenated oil: popcorn shrimp and frozen pizzas

Sodium Nitrite

Some processed meats may contain sodium nitrites to help the meat appear a pretty pink. Nitrites are used to inhibit botulism-causing bacteria but once ingested it can fuse with amino acids to form nitrosamines which are powerful carcinogenic compounds, though, manufacturers are now attempting to decrease that risk by adding ascorbic and erythorbic acids (vitamin C). Nonetheless, limit your intake whenever possible.

Food(s) which may have sodium nitrite: bacon and hot dogs

Caramel Coloring

This additive wouldn't be dangerous if made the old-fashioned way using sugar and on top of a stove. Unfortunately, the food industry uses a different method—they treat sugar with ammonia, possibly producing nasty carcinogens. High levels of caramel coloring can be found in colas and a Center for Science in the Public Interest report stated there are roughly 15,000 cancers in the U.S. reported annually. May just be another good reason to stop drinking sodas?

Item(s) which may have caramel coloring: colas

Castoreum

Castoreum is used to flavor food and is referred to as a "natural ingredient." Even though it isn't harmful, you're not going to like where it comes from. Castoreum comes from beavers' castor sacs, or anal scent glands. Makes you want to gag, I know! Beavers mark their territory by spraying this musky scent from their anal glands. Get a load of this: over 1,000 pounds of this unsavory ingredient is used annually by food manufacturers to flavor foods. Yuck!

Food(s) which may have castoreum: any food claiming "natural ingredients"

Food Dyes

Sugary cereals and fruit-flavored candies contain artificial dyes and flavorings to suggest a relationship with "nature." Manufacturers use food dyes to enhance the lifeless colors of their product(s). Bad news is there are hues which have been linked to serious ailments. A *Journal of Pediatrics* study linked Yellow 5 to hyperactivity in children, Canadian researchers found Yellow 6 and Red 40 to be contaminated with known carcinogens, and Red 3 is known to cause tumors. Please, as much as possible, avoid foods and beverages using dyes.

Food(s) which may have food dyes: sugary cereals, gelatin desserts

Hydrolyzed Vegetable Protein

Hydrolyzed vegetable protein is a plant protein that has been chemically broken down into amino acids and is used to enhance foods. Trouble is that when one of the amino acids, called glutamic acid, releases free glutamate and joins with free sodium in your body, they can form monosodium glutamate (MSG). MSG has been known to cause nausea and headaches. The FDA requires manufacturers to label their products when MSG is added to their product(s). However, if it occurs as a byproduct, the FDA allows it to go unrecognized.

Food(s) which may have hydrolyzed vegetable protein: hot dogs, soups/stews/chili, sauces and/or gravies

8

INTOLERANCES AND ALLERGIES

Food allergies and intolerances are very common and can cause really un-fun symptoms such as skin rashes, stomach cramps, diarrhea, tiredness and more. I, unfortunately, have developed all kinds of food allergies.

YOU KNOW, EVERYTHING IN MODERATION

I never had food allergies until I was an adult. Actually, my first food allergy became evident in high school. Every Friday evening my mom would have shrimp cocktail for me as a treat. I believe she spoiled me with this weekly treat because she and my dad would go out for dinner and I think she felt badly that I was left home alone, eating alone. The gift of shrimp cocktail worked, I felt *the love*. Who doesn't love shellfish? Anyway, sadly, it turns out I was having too much of a good thing. I ended up allergic to all shellfish.

Here's what happened. One evening after eating out at The Red Lobster with my high school sweetheart, Tommy, I ended up with terrible stomach cramps and welts all over my body. This was an allergic reaction I had never experienced before, and it was all due to food. I didn't just have hives. Well, they started out as extremely itchy hives but then the hives grew into golf-ball size welts! It was really scary. I looked like an alien. Tommy rushed me to the emergency room. The ER doctors asked me what I had eaten for dinner and I told them shellfish. They said, "That's it." Never before had I been allergic to food. They also told me, "You might not make it to the emergency room in time, the next time." Hence, the reason I now have my EpiPen® close by and I know I have to always pay attention to what is being served to make sure shellfish isn't hidden in dips, etc. Here's something one might not know: there are restaurants which deep-fry shrimp and they use the same oil to deep-fry potatoes to make their French fries. It could be actually deadly! So, if you have an allergy to shellfish, or you know someone else who does, please be aware of this.

The same thing happened to me with peanut butter, wheat bread, pasta, crackers and strawberries. I would get on these stretches of loving too much of one kind of food. By over-indulging in the foods I loved, I became allergic to them. I mention this to you to instill the importance of everything in moderation and to challenge you to please pay attention to any signs or symptoms coming from your body. It may be flashing signals that some foods or beverages are not agreeing with your body.

Again, the most common food allergies/intolerances are gluten and dairy but some may be allergic to things like corn, eggs, soy, peanuts and citrus.

BLOOD TYPES AND INTOLERANCES

Did you know that your blood type could also play a part in which foods to avoid for any possible allergy or intolerance. Do you know which blood type you are? There's O, A, B and AB. Well, get a load of these findings.

Blood Type O is the oldest blood type of all, dating back to 30,000 BC. Folks who have the O blood type can have an intolerance to corn and wheat. This means for those of you with the O blood type, you may need to stay away from baked goods. Good news, though. Those of you with O do well eating meat. It makes sense if you think about what individuals had to do to survive back then, they hunted and ate, primarily, meat, this was back in the day of hunters and gatherers, right? So, this blood type does well with a diet high in protein.

Blood Type A began around 25,000 BC this is when communities started growing their food, just think of "A" for agriculture. Folks with the A blood type do well on a vegetarian-type daily diet. They have strong, lean bodies due to the healthy grains they are eating but one could have an issue with meat, dairy and even some beans, such as soybeans.

Have you heard folks say, "A person's DNA can't be changed"? Well, blood types have evolved over the centuries and blood is DNA. So don't believe you're stuck with your family's poor-health DNA. If you can make healthier choices and possibly change your outcome in order to live a long, happy, healthy life—wouldn't you? You betcha!

Nonetheless, then around 15,000 BC the evolution of the Blood Type B came to be. This group of individuals mainly lived in a climate where it was too cold to hunt and fish. Thus,

they turned to their farm animals to enjoy eggs and they created things like cheese, yogurt, milk, etc., to thrive and survive
on. Those with B blood can typically enjoy dairy foods and
beverages without any issues but might need to steer clear of
peanuts and wheat; guess my blood type in light of my food
allergies. Yep, I'm B.

Last but not least, the Blood Type AB is the most recently
evolved blood type, evolving around 2500 BC. This group
does well on a real mixture of foods but again may have a
challenge with things like corn or buckwheat.

So find out your blood type and continue to pay attention to
how you feel when you eat certain foods or drink certain beverages. In this chapter, I'll skim over some possible allergies and
food intolerances, but I am not going to go into great detail
on specific allergies and intolerances because this book would
double in size but I encourage you to pay attention to when
you feel crummy after eating/drinking. Get tested by an allergist, if need be, to rule out whether or not you have an issue.

DAIRY-FREE AND/OR GLUTEN-FREE
The most common food allergies are gluten and dairy. Do
you know anyone who has to be gluten-free or dairy-free
when eating/drinking? I am 100% Finnish (though born here
in the U.S.) and did you know that the Finnish have the highest percentage of celiac disease than any other nationality?
I've been told the McDonalds restaurants in Finland serve all
of their burgers and sandwiches on gluten-free buns. Well,
I've never been tested for celiac disease but I do have an
intolerance to wheat so I stay clear of it the best I can. Every
great once in a while I will opt to have toast or a sandwich

but when I do my belly ends up all bloated and gassy. Does that ever happen to you after you've had certain foods or beverages? Again, this is a great time to journal what you've had so that you can keep track of those times when things didn't agree with you.

MILK—IT IS UP IN THE AIR

Whether or not one should drink milk is a personal preference. If you enjoy it and it agrees with your body then by all means keep on drinking it. I personally think FairLife™ is a wonderful brand. FairLife™ has 50% more calcium and contains less sugar than other milks on the market. Have you ever tried FairLife™'s chocolate milk? It is off-the-charts! But remember, in moderation.

There is a lot to consider when it comes to milk. Is low-fat healthier than whole milk? Should it be pasteurized or is raw better? Is organic necessary and really the best?

If you are up in the air about it, let me share the following with you about milk . . .

ORGANIC MILK

Pro:

- High in beta carotene, omega-3 and vitamin E
- Cows are not eating GMO feed
- No synthetic-hormones, chemical fertilizers, toxic pesticides and no antibiotics
- Cows get to romp around on outdoor pastures

Con:

- Naturally-occurring growth hormones can be present
- If heated to 280° F beneficial bacteria can be killed off

NON-ORGANIC MILK

Pro:

- Harmful bacteria in non-organic milk can be treated with antibiotics

Con:

- Synthetic contaminants, growth hormones and pesticides
- Possibility of cows dining on GMO feed

GRASS FED COWS

Pro:

- High in omega-3 and vitamin D3
- It's kind for dairy farmers to be feeding their cows grass
- Can contain higher CLA (conjugated linoleic acid) which can aid in losing weight and can help protect your "ticker", your heart

Con (for dairy farmers):

- May need to invest in more pasture acreage
- Can get frustrating with cows needing more grazing time

LOW-FAT/FAT-FREE/SKIM MILK

Pro:

- Fewer calories
- Less saturated fats

Con:

- Your body may become low in vitamins A and D

FULL-FAT/WHOLE MILK

Pro:

- Can help your digestive system digest fat-soluble vitamins

Con:

- High in calories (for those of you needing to slim down)
- High in saturated fat (as you know, stay clear of these fats)

RAW MILK

Pro:

- Those who are lactose intolerant may find raw milk with the enzyme lipase, easier to digest
- Tastes AWESOME
- Has good-for-you bacteria
- Vitamins and minerals are present naturally

Con:

- Doesn't last long, only about a week in the frig
- You may get sick if there are pathogens present
- Not easy to buy, so many states prohibit the sale of raw milk

PROCESSED MILK

Pro:

- Pathogens/bacteria are killed off
- Fortified with vitamins A and D, which helps with calcium absorption

Con:

- Possibility of some good-for-you bacteria to be killed off
- Possibility of destroying enzymes, vitamins and minerals

BENEFITS OF DRINKING MILK

Okay, now that you know a little bit more about milk, I don't want it to sound so negative. For those of you who love it and if it is working well for you, keep on drinking it. Let's talk about the benefits. Milk is good for your bones. It is high in calcium, protein, vitamin D, magnesium, potassium and phosphorus. Remember, potassium is good for muscle cramps too.

Milk that is processed in the United States is fortified with 100 IU of vitamin D per serving. Some recommend you drink three glasses per day. What is your preference?

If you find yourself getting hungry between meals, try drinking a glass of milk with each meal. The protein in milk will help you feel fuller longer. For those of you who are always starving, milk can be a great thing to have before a game and between tournament games.

It is said that milk is kind to diabetics because the sugar (lactose) in milk breaks down nice and slowly—thus no spike in one's blood sugar. If you're diabetic ask your doctor his/her opinion.

SOME REASONS TO CONSIDER NOT DRINKING MILK

It is thought that milk can weaken your bones due to its high levels of vitamin A.

Folks who are lactose intolerant may face the unpleasant issue of diarrhea. If you are faced with constant diarrhea, you could end up with serious deficiencies in vitamins and minerals.

So, it's your choice whether or not to drink milk. What is your body telling you after you've been drinking milk. You decide. Remember, you are in control.

GRAINS (I.E. WHEAT)

Here again, this all depends upon the individual. For those of you who *do not* have an allergy or an intolerance, enjoy all of the wonderful, good-for-you grains out there. And, what am I going to recommend to you, once again? Keep a note, journal how you feel after you've eaten whole grains.

Grains can give you loads of energy. It's energy which will stick with you for extended periods of time because grains are absorbed nice and slowly by your body. If you can tolerate whole grains, you will be rewarded with a fantastically fit figure, a lean, strong physique.

Plus, more importantly, whole grains are a wonderful source of the following nutrients:

- Dietary fiber
- E and B-complex vitamins
- Enzymes

Here is a list of great grains for you to dine on:

- Oatmeal (rolled or, preferably, steel cut)
- Brown rice
- Wild rice
- Quinoa
- Couscous
- Pita bread
- Millet
- Wheat
- Pasta
- Dark breads/whole-grain breads
- Buckwheat
- Kasha
- *Even* . . . Beer! (legal-aged drinking individuals, ONLY!)

POSSIBLE ISSUES WITH GLUTEN

Follow your gut. What is it that I keep telling you? Take note.

Journal. Ask yourself, after eating grains, how did I feel? Did you find yourself suffering from any of these symptoms:

- Migraines/headaches
- Tiredness/fatigue
- Grumpy mood swings/irritable as a "wet hen"
- Diarrhea/excessive gassiness

What is possibly happening for so many folks is that they are developing an intolerance to the protein found in grains. This protein is known as gluten. Where gluten can be present:

- Wheat
- Rye
- Barley
- Oats (contaminated oats)

The trouble with gluten is that it can eat away at the little villi that is lining your intestines. Villi are the important little buggers which help pull nutrients into your bloodstream. When one's villi are killed off in the small intestine, malnutrition can be a very serious consequence.

Before I go too deeply into the subject, please note that having celiac disease can be very serious, even deadly. This is an area where I want to refer you to the experts.

I picked up the wonderful book "The G Free Diet" by Elisabeth Hasselbeck (once a cohost of *The View)* to become better educated on whether or not I needed to cut out wheat from my diet, basically go gluten-free.

I, personally, experienced horrible symptoms when I ingested too much wheat bread, pasta, cereals and crackers. I developed severe itchiness on my knees and elbows. My elbows and knees would become bloody because I scratched them so feverishly due to the intense itchiness. Thus, I now choose to live a pretty gluten-free lifestyle. The discomfort I endured was not worth the foods I was eating.

The good news is that there are a lot of gluten-free products available in the stores today. One of my favorite is Crunchmaster® Multi-Grain Crackers; give them a try. I bet you'll love them more than other crackers found at the store which contain gluten.

DO YOU HAVE AN ALLERGY OR INTOLERANCE? TRY AN ELIMINATION DIET

As you know, it's your choice. You get to decide what you want to put into your body. Would you like to discover whether or not you have an allergy or an intolerance to certain foods/beverages? I suggest you try an elimination diet. For instance, don't eat any baked goods or avoid dairy products for a week or two; write down how you were feeling emotionally, physically and mentally. Then re-introduce those foods and/or beverages back into your daily diet. Do you find yourself feeling poorly again? Could be you have an intolerance or an allergy. I suggest you also reach out and talk to your doctor if you're experiencing problems with certain foods and beverages. Get tested by an allergist and in severe cases you may want to get tested for the celiac gene. Your body is your best barometer. Remember, your body will give you signals when things aren't right.

9 | NUTRITIONAL TIDBITS

Keep in mind that this particular chapter may be a bit boring or you might find it so fascinating you won't be able to put the book down. Either way, at least you can always return to this chapter, if and when you're curious as to what are the health benefits of certain foods/beverages you come across.

I will say, though, that I am pretty sure you're going to be amazed at how wonderful food is and how many are so good for you. WARNING: You may become very hungry and thirsty for healthy foods and beverages.

Superfoods: Let's begin with superfoods! Have you heard of micro- and phytonutrients? Well, they are an essential part of what your body needs to function at its best and they can be found in superfoods. When you incorporate superfoods into your daily diet you will experience better digestion, your muscles will become stronger and any injury you have will heal more quickly. Here is a list of some superfoods:

- Acai

- Apples
- Beets
- Blueberries
- Broccoli
- Carrots
- Cranberries
- Goji berries
- Kale
- Pomegranates
- Spinach

Not a huge fan of some of those foods? I have a solution. I strongly encourage my clients to get all of the nutrients they need from whole foods and beverages but sometimes that's not so easy to do, especially if you're not a fan of things like broccoli. And, if you're not a fan of broccoli, don't feel bad. What many folks don't know is that the reason so many of us don't like broccoli is because it does not agree with our body. It's true. Individuals who have a body which is naturally high in sulfur will reject foods which are high in sulfur and broccoli is one of them. So, parents, back off on the broccoli if your "cub" can't stand the taste of it. It's not agreeing with your child's body chemistry.

As I mentioned, I do have a solution to help you incorporate all of the above superfoods into one meal. No, no, no, I'm not suggesting you buy and eat all of the above in one sitting, I'm suggesting you invest in Skoop™. Here's the skinny:

Skoop™: Superfoods done easy! Scoop™ has all of the above-mentioned organic fruits and vegetables in one easy scoop. It's an amazing probiotic. Probiotics help you poop. There are 5 grams of dietary fiber in one scoop from a beautiful blend of organic gum acacia, flaxseed and chia. The enzymes in Skoop™ will give you lots of energy. It's low in sugar. It's gluten free! And, being chockfull of amino acids, it will help you build muscle. With its alkalizing minerals it helps bring your Ph level to an alkaline state versus acidic. An alkaline body keeps cold and flu away; so important to not miss a game or practice, right? You betcha!

For the FDA panel info on Skoop™, please visit: http://coachloves.healthyskoop.com

Back to the basics on all of the wonderful foods and beverages out there for you. As you are well aware reading labels is imperative to understanding what exactly you're putting into your body. Though I'm sure you're saying to yourself, "Roxanne, you're always promoting nothing but whole foods. Nothing in a package. Well, where's the nutritional label on an apple? Or a banana?" Not to worry. I have taken the necessary steps to seek high and low to give you nutritional information on all kinds of wonderful foods, superfoods and beverages. I am hoping to introduce you to foods you may never think of eating—foods and beverages to nourish your body so you can perform like you've never performed before on and off ice.

Acai: Superfood! Acai (ah-sigh-EE) berries are harvested from acai palm trees, native to South America rain forests. Acai berries are helpful for arthritis, cancer, weight loss, high cholesterol, erectile dysfunction, detoxification and improved health in general. 100 gm: calories: 70; fat: 5g; sodium: 10mg; carbs: 4g [2g dietary fiber, 2g sugars]; protein: 1g; Vitamin A: 15%; Vitamin C: 0%; Calcium: 2%; Iron 0%. .

Almonds: May lower your LDL-cholesterol, your risk of heart disease and protect you against diabetes. Plus, the healthy fats in almonds may help you lose weight (if need be). Almonds contain manganese, copper and riboflavin; thus they can help with your energy level. Folks who consume almonds also had a lower chance of developing gallstones. 1 cup raw: calories: 546; fat: 47g; sodium: 1mg; carbs: 21g [12g dietary fiber, 4g sugars]; protein: 20g; Vitamin A: 0%; Vitamin C: 0%; Calcium: 25%; Iron: 20%.

Apples: Superfood! Full of phyto-nutrients and anti-oxidants promoting growth, development, and overall wellness. Rich in dietary fiber, preventing absorption of bad cholesterol in the gut and saves the mucous membrane in your colon from toxic substances. Apples are a good source of B-complex vitamins such as riboflavin, thiamin, and pyridoxine (vitamin B-6) and has a small amount of minerals like potassium which helps control heart rate and blood pressure. 1 cup raw, chopped: calories: 65; fat: 0g; sodium: 1mg; carbs: 17g [3g dietary fiber, 13g sugars]; protein: 0g; Vitamin A: 1%; Vitamin C: 10%; Calcium: 1%; Iron 1%. Storage: To extend the life of apples put them in a plastic bag in your refrigerator. When apples are kept at room temperature they will ripen ten times faster than an apple kept at 32°F.

Bananas: During your game, between periods, gobble down a banana to help boost your brain power/concentration.

Bananas contain three natural sugars—sucrose, fructose and glucose combined with fiber. A banana gives an instant, sustained and substantial boost of energy. Research has proven that just two bananas provide enough energy for a strenuous 90-minute workout. No wonder the banana is the number one fruit with the world's leading athletes. But energy isn't the only way a banana can help us keep fit. It can also help overcome or prevent a substantial number of illnesses and conditions, making it a must to add to our daily diet.

If you're feeling low, feeling a little depressed, eat a banana. Bananas contain tryptophan, a type of protein that the body converts into serotonin, known to make you relax, improve your mood and generally make you feel happier. Vitamin B6, found in bananas, helps to regulate blood glucose levels, which can affect your mood. Also, high in iron, bananas can stimulate the production of hemoglobin in the blood and so helps in cases of anemia (blood low in iron).

Bananas are extremely high in potassium yet low in salt, making them perfect to beat blood pressure. So much so, the U.S. Food and Drug Administration has just allowed the banana industry to make official claims for the fruit's ability to reduce the risk of blood pressure and stroke.

If you're having a challenge going to the bathroom (particularly when you're traveling for tournaments) have a banana as a natural laxative. You will restore normal bowel action.

Are you experiencing heartburn when having to dine out during hockey tournaments? Sometimes you have no choice because of limited healthy options on restaurant menus but if you end up with heartburn you can eat a banana. It has a natural antacid effect.

If you're away at a wonderful hockey camp this summer and end up with mosquito bites all over try rubbing the affected area with the inside of a banana skin. It can help reduce swelling and irritation.

Feeling a little nervous before your game? Bananas help calm the nerves because they're high in vitamin B6.

The banana versus the apple . . . a banana has four times the protein, twice as much complex carbohydrates, three times the phosphorus, five times the vitamin A and iron, twice the other vitamins and minerals, and is richer in potassium.

1 cup raw: calories: 200; fat: 1g; sodium: 2mg; carbs: 51g [6g dietary fiber, 28g sugars]; protein: 2g; Vitamin A: 3%; Vitamin C: 33%; Calcium: 1%; Iron 3%. Storage: Do not refrigerate bananas (unless you want them frozen for smoothies). To speed up the ripening of green bananas, put them in a bag and place in a warm spot, like on top of the refrigerator.

TIP: Buy bananas in bulk, it's cheaper. Peel each banana and place them all into a Ziploc™ freezer bag and keep in the freezer. Pull out a banana from the freezer whenever you want to make a smoothie. Simply place the frozen banana into your Vitamix™, along with your other ingredients, blend and enjoy!

Beets: Superfood! Highly nutritious, root vegetable. You can eat both the root and the green tops. The dark, red-purple pigment is full of antioxidants which offers protection against coronary artery disease, stroke; can lower cholesterol levels; and has anti-aging effects. 1 cup raw: calories: 8; fat: 0g; sodium: 86mg; carbs: 2g [1g dietary fiber, 0g sugars]; protein: 1g; Vitamin A: 48%; Vitamin C: 19%; Calcium: 4%; Iron: 5%.

Blueberries: Superfood! Rich in pro-anthocyanin, natural pigment anti-oxidants. Attributed to longevity and wellness. 1 cup raw: calories: 84; fat: 0g; sodium: 1mg; carbs: 21g [4g dietary fiber, 15g sugars]; protein: 1g; Vitamin A: 2%; Vitamin C: 24%; Calcium: 1%; Iron: 2%.

Broccoli: Superfood! Can help prevent cancer, helps keep your immune system strong, lowers your blood pressure, promotes healthy heart, bones and eyes. 1 cup raw, chopped: calories: 31; fat: 0g; sodium: 30mg; carbs: 6g [2g dietary fiber, 2g sugars]; protein: 3g; Vitamin A: 11%; Vitamin C: 135%; Calcium: 4%; Iron: 4%. Storage: Can be stored for up to three days in the vegetable crisper drawer of your refrigerator. To refresh and bring back broccoli's bright green color put it in ice water.

Brown Rice: FYI, unlike white rice, brown rice has all its bran layers intact. Thus, its layers of bran protect all of its nutrients and fatty acids. Brown rice contains the highest amounts of B vitamins, iron, vitamin E, amino acids, and linoleic acid. It is high in fiber, low in sodium, and is composed of 80% complex carbohydrates. Brown rice promotes good digestion, quenches thirst and helps to balance blood sugar. If you're experiencing mood swings, brown rice can help (your teammates, family and friends will be grateful). 1 cup raw, long-grain, cooked: calories: 216; fat: 2g; sodium: 10mg; carbs: 45g [4g dietary fiber, 1g sugars]; protein: 5g; Vitamin A: 0%; Vitamin C: 0%; Calcium: 2%; Iron: 5%.

Carrots with Tops: Superfood! Strengthens your immune system and helps destroy pre-cancerous cells. 1 large: calories: 5; fat: 0g; sodium: 12mg; carbs: 1g [0g dietary fiber, 1g sugars]; protein: 0g; Vitamin A: 41%; Vitamin C: 1%; Calcium: 0%; Iron: 1%. Storage: Remove green tops, rinse, drain and place in plastic bags. By storing them at the high-humidity level in the crisper drawer and the coldest section of the refrigerator they can last several months before spoiling.

Cauliflower: Known to fight cancer with its sulfur compound, sulforaphane, it has been shown to slow tumor growth by killing off cancer stem cells. Mix cauliflower and the spice curcumin (found in turmeric) to help prevent and treat prostate cancer. Labs done with rats and mice found cauliflower to inhibit the development of cancer in the lung, liver, breast, bladder, stomach and colon. Boosts a healthy heart by improving blood pressure and kidney function. It's an anti-Inflammatory; inflammation damage is linked to cancer and other diseases. It's overflowing in vitamins and minerals: vitamin K, protein, thiamin, riboflavin, niacin, magnesium, phosphorus, fiber, vitamin B6, folate, pantothenic acid, potassium, and manganese. Boosts your brain: cognitive functions, improved learning and memory. Detoxifies. It's a great source of dietary fiber, plus, it protect the lining of your stomach. 1 cup raw, chopped: calories: 25; fat: 0g; sodium: 30mg; carbs: 5g [3g dietary fiber, 2g sugars]; protein: 2g; Vitamin A: 0%; Vitamin C: 7%; Calcium: 2%; Iron: 2%. Storage: Can be stored for up to three days in the vegetable crisper drawer of your refrigerator.

Celery: Another anti-inflammatory and chockfull of antioxidants protecting against unwanted oxygen damage to cells, blood vessels and your organ systems. 1 cup raw: calories: 18; fat: 0g; sodium: 88mg; carbs: 4g [2g dietary fiber, 2g sugars]; protein: 1g; Vitamin A: 10%; Vitamin C: 6%; Calcium: 4%; Iron: 1%. Storage: Trim off the base, rinse and remove leaves and discard any ribs which are damaged or bruised. Wrap with a paper towel and put it in a plastic bag in the crisper drawer. Celery will last about two weeks.

Cherries: Superfood! Challenges with arthritis or gout? Eat some cherries. They also help prevent memory loss. Reduces the risk of heart disease. 1 cup raw: calories: 77; fat: 0g; sodium: 5mg; carbs: 19g (2g dietary fiber, 13g sugars]; protein: 2g; Vitamin A: 40%, Vitamin C: 26%; Calcium: 2%, Iron: 3%.

Chia Seeds: Chia seeds are believed to be an energy booster. They are chockfull of carbs, protein, healthy omega-3s, fiber, calcium, vitamins, minerals and antioxidants. 2 tablespoons: calories: 139; fat: 9g; carbs: 12g (11g dietary fiber); protein: 4g. Sprinkle on your yogurt, oatmeal and in your smoothies.

Coconut Oil: Coconut oil can boost thyroid function, resulting in an increase in metabolism, energy and endurance. It helps fight off viruses, bacteria, yeast, fungus and candida. It positively affects blood sugar, thus, improving insulin use within the body. It helps with digestion and promotes absorption of fat-soluble vitamins. The lauric acid in coconut oil increases good cholesterol (HDL). Coconut oil can help keep weight balanced and it can help with aging, as it is a antioxidant. Oxidation is considered a major contributor to cardiovascular problems and skin aging. It is a wonderful moisturizer for your hair and skin. It has good amounts of the antioxidant vitamin E, too. Use coconut oil in both baked goods and when cooking vegetables, like kale. To make your oatmeal more creamy, add coconut oil. It can withstand heat, thus making it a terrific cooking oil. Use daily, about one to two tablespoons a day can be beneficial.

Collards: Has the ability to lower one's cholesterol and helps lower cancer risk by detoxing your system and with its anti-inflammatory properties. 1 cup raw: calories: 11; fat: 0g; sodium: 7mg; carbs: 2g [1g dietary fiber, 0g sugars]; protein: 1g; Vitamin A: 48%; Vitamin C: 21%; Calcium: 5%; Iron: 0%. Storage: Wrap unwashed greens up in dampened paper towels and place into a plastic bag. When kept in the crisper drawer of the refrigerator it can last for up to five days.

Corn: Yellow corn is a high-carotenoid food and is heavily concentrated in the antioxidants lutein and zeaxanthin. It is also a good source of fiber supporting healthy bacteria in our large intestine, thus, lowering risk of cancer in your colon. No better time than summer to enjoy fresh corn-on-the-cob from the farmer's market! 1 cup raw: calories: 132; fat: 2g; sodium: 23mg; carbs: 29g [4g dietary fiber, 5g sugars]; protein: 5g; Vitamin A: 0%; Vitamin C: 17%; Calcium: 0%; Iron: 4%. Storage: If it can't be eaten right away, store in the refrigerator in plastic bags with the husks still on; it will last for a few days when stored this way.

Cranberries: Superfood! Cranberries and cranberry juice can help prevent urinary tract infections (UTIs) and stomach bacteria (*Helicobacter pylori*). Plus, preliminary studies also show cranberries may protect you from stomach ulcers. Anthocyanins, in water-harvested cranberries, can provide you with healthy benefits of antioxidant and anti-inflammatory properties. Studies have shown that whole cranberries protect your cardiovascular system and your liver. Scientists believe cranberries have cancer-preventive benefits with regard to breast, colon, lung, and prostate cancers. 1 cup raw: calories: 46; fat: 0.1g; sodium: 2mg; carbs: 12g [4g dietary fiber, 4g sugars]; protein: 0.4g; Vitamin A: 1%; Vitamin C: 22%; Calcium: 0%; Iron: 1%.

Flaxseed: Some folks believe flaxseed is *the* most powerful plant food on this earth. It is believed that it may help reduce your risk of diabetes, cardiovascular/heart disease, stroke and even cancer. Flaxseed contains the essential fatty acid,

Omega-3, which is a super good fat for your heart. And, it contains lignans, a plant estrogen and an awesome antioxidant. Flaxseed is both a soluble and insoluble fiber. Sprinkle flaxseed on your oatmeal or throw it in your smoothies, especially helpful if you have a hard time pooping when you're traveling for tournaments. Some folks get bound up when they can't use their own bathroom at home.

Goji Berries: Superfood! Loaded with beta-carotene, helping to promote healthy skin. Goji berries have been known to help boost the immune system. An excellent source of vitamin C, thus, can help reduce cold symptoms. Overall, a terrific source of antioxidants and loaded with fiber. 1/4 cup raw: calories: 100; fat: 1g; sodium: 90mg; carbs: 19g [2g dietary fiber, 15g sugars]; protein: 4g; Vitamin A: 30%; Vitamin C: 10%; Calcium: 2%; Iron: 20%.

Grapes: Red, seedless grapes with their phytonutrients and resveratrol are believed to play a part in longevity. 1 cup raw: calories: 104; fat: 0g; sodium: 3mg; carbs: 27g [1g dietary fiber, 23g sugars]; protein: 1g; Vitamin A: 2%; Vitamin C: 27%; Calcium: 2%; Iron: 3%. Storage: Remove spoiled grapes and refrigerate; they will keep up to a week. TIP: Freeze grapes, which tastes wonderfully cool and refreshing during the summer; by freezing them, they can last up to three months.

Green Beans: Green beans have carotenoids, antioxidants and flavonoids and the mineral silicon which is very important for bone health and formation of connective tissue. 1 cup raw: calories: 34; fat: 0g; sodium: 7mg; carbs: 8g [4g dietary fiber, 2g sugars]; protein: 2g; Vitamin A: 15%; Vitamin C: 30%; Calcium: 4%; Iron: 6%. Storage: By putting your fresh green beans in a plastic bag (perforated) or paper bag, they can be stored for up to five days in the refrigerator crisper.

Guavas: Superfood! Can't poop or are you faced with miserable diarrhea? Eat some guava, great source of fiber and minerals. Guava is known to help fight fevers. Prevents heart disease and cancer. Skin issues, too. 1 cup raw: calories: 112; fat: 2g; sodium: 3mg; carbs: 24g [9g dietary fiber, 15g sugars]; protein: 4g; Vitamin A: 21%; Vitamin C: 628%; Calcium: 3%; Iron: 2%.

Kale: Superfood! Can help prevent cancer, helps keep your immune system strong, lowers your blood pressure, promotes healthy heart, bones and eyes. 1 cup chopped: calories: 33; fat: 0g; sodium: 29mg; carbs: 7g [1g dietary fiber, 6g sugars]: protein: 2g; Vitamin A: 206%; Vitamin C: 134%; Calcium: 9%; Iron: 6%.

Kiwi: Superfood! Kiwi can help prevent asthma. Helps control sugar levels, which is great for diabetics. Kiwi is also known for helping curb a nasty cough. 1 cup raw: calories: 108; fat: 1g; sodium: 5mg; carbs: 26g [5g dietary fiber, 16g sugars]; protein: 2g; Vitamin A: 3%; Vitamin C: 273%; Calcium: 6%; Iron 3%. To ripen, keep at room temperature but away from heat/direct sunlight for a few days to a week. Once ripe, keep away from other fruits to avoid over-ripening; should keep for about one to two weeks.

Kombucha: An ancient Chinese elixir. Health benefits are said to prevent and fight cancer, arthritis, and other degenerative diseases. It is made with sweetened tea and a bacteria and yeast called SCOBY. It is high in nutrients such as B-vitamins, antioxidants and glucaric acids. It helps detoxify your liver.

Kombucha contains glucosamines, a nice treatment for all forms of arthritis. It aids in digestion and creates a healthy gut. Kombucha is a probiotic beverage. It also helps with mental clarity and mood stability and is noted for reducing or eliminating the symptoms of fibromyalgia, depression, anxiety, etc. Not to mention the wonderful immune boosting properties. Plus, Kombucha can increase one's energy levels.

Lettuce: By adding salads to your daily diet, lettuce is known to help prevent osteoporosis, anemia (iron deficiency), and is believed to help protect you against cardiovascular diseases, Alzheimer's and cancers. 1 cup shredded, raw: calories: 10; fat: 0g; sodium: 7mg; carbs: 2g [1g dietary fiber, 1g sugars]; protein: 1g; Vitamin A: 7%; Vitamin C: 3%; Calcium: 1%; Iron: 2%. Storage: Place unwashed leaves in a plastic bag with a single sheet of paper towel and put in crisper drawer; should keep for up to five days. Do not store lettuce near fruits because they can cause the lettuce to turn brown.

Lignans: A plant estrogen and great antioxidant. Studies have been done and results have shown that women who consumed lignans had a lower BMI (body mass index) than those who didn't, plus, they had lower glucose (sugar in their blood) numbers. Lignans may also lower the risk of breast and prostate cancer and help prevent hair loss.

Macronutrients: Nutrients found in protein, carbs and fats.

Mangoes: Mangoes are rich in fiber, vitamins, minerals, flavonoids and antioxidants. They are found to protect against colon, breast, leukemia, prostate and breast cancers. With a high level of vitamin A, mangoes help you maintain healthy mucus membranes and skin. A good source of potassium, important for cell and body fluids, which helps control heart rate and blood pressure. A good source of vitamin-B6, vitamins C and E, plus, copper which is required for the production of red blood cells. 1 cup raw: calories: 107; fat: 0g; sodium: 3mg; carbs: 28g [3g dietary fiber, 24g sugars]; protein: 1g; Vitamin A: 25%; Vitamin C: 76%; Calcium: 2%; Iron: 1%. Storage: To ripen keep at a cool room temp for a few days. To speed up the process put two mangoes or another fruit such as an apple or banana in a paper bag; Once ripe they can keep up to two to three days in the refrigerator.

Melons: An excellent source of Vitamin A and a powerful anti-oxidant and essential for healthy vision, mucus membranes and skin. Consumption of melons can help protect you from lung, colon, prostate, breast, endometrial and pancreatic cancers. Instead of a sports drink, eat melon. A moderate source of electrolytes and potassium. Potassium can protect you from stroke and coronary heart diseases. Their antioxidants fight against infectious agents and scavenge harmful oxygen-free radicals. 1 cup raw: calories: 64; fat: 0g; sodium: 32mg; carbs: 16g [1g dietary fiber, 14g sugars]; protein: 1g; Vitamin A: 2%; Vitamin C: 53%; Calcium: 1%; Iron: 2%. Storage: Ripe melons (whole or cut) can be stored for three days in the refrigerator. Cut melons need to be wrapped tightly in plastic. If you leave the seeds inside a cut melon it will help keep it moist until ready to eat.

Micronutrients: Critical vitamins and minerals essential for the body.

Oatmeal: Lowers cholesterol levels, reduces the risk of high blood pressure and heart attack, lowers risk of heart failure. Enhances your immune system. Stabilizes your blood sugar; keeps your blood sugar levels under control.

Can protect you from developing breast cancer (keep in mind that men get breast cancer too; this isn't just for the female player). Oatmeal has been known to help with protecting kids from asthma. *Caution:* However, wheat, is a common food allergen, which may trigger asthma. Eating whole grain oats can protect against atherosclerosis, ischemic stroke, diabetes, insulin resistance, obesity, and premature death. A new study published in the *American Journal of Clinical Nutrition* explains the likely reasons behind these findings and recommends at least 3 servings of whole grains should be eaten daily. 1 cup: 200 calories; 9g carbs; 7g fiber; 1g of iron. Enjoy with fruit or make it savory by adding sautéed spinach, scrambled egg whites and hot sauce on top. For added energy and a real boost, sprinkle some Skoop™ on top of your oatmeal to give your body the nutrients it's craving or missing.

Onions: Onions have important nutrients and health-promoting phytochemicals. They are high in vitamin C, calcium, iron and folic acid. Onions are high in fiber and have a high protein quality. Plus, they are low in sodium and contain zero fat. Antioxidants found in onions may delay or slow the oxidative damage to cells and body tissue. Onions may help prevent gastric ulcers. They have the potential to decrease the possibility of osteoporosis and may even protect against cataracts, cardiovascular disease, cancer of the breast, colon, ovarian, lung and bladder. 1 cup raw: calories: 64; fat: 0g; sodium: 6mg; carbs: 15g [3g dietary fiber, 7g sugars]; protein: 2g; Vitamin A: 0%; Vitamin C: 20%; Calcium: 4%; Iron: 2%. Storage: Keep onions in a dry and dark, well-ventilated place; do not refrigerate.

Oranges: Oranges contain phytonutrients and are an excellent source of vitamin C, reducing your risk of colon cancer, asthma, osteoarthritis, rheumatoid arthritis, heart disease, and stroke. Studies have shown that consuming citrus can help prevent Alzheimer's disease and cognitive impairment, Parkinson's disease, macular degeneration, diabetes, gallstones, multiple sclerosis, cholera, gingivitis, optimal lung function, cataracts, ulcerative colitis and Crohn's disease. Oranges have the potential to lower cholesterol levels, too. They are a wonderful source of fiber reducing constipation or diarrhea (IBS—irritable bowel syndrome).

They may even prevent kidney stones. Last, but not least, oranges can help your respiratory system. 1 cup raw: calories: 85; fat: 0g; sodium: 0mg; carbs: 21g [4g dietary fiber, 17g sugars]; protein: 1g; Vitamin A: 8%; Vitamin C: 139%; Calcium: 8%; Iron: 1%. Storage: Keep oranges in a cool place, not in the refrigerator. Try to eat them within a few days. If you need to keep them longer, put them in a plastic bag in the vegetable crisper of the refrigerator.

Pears: Please don't peel your pear, the skin contains anti-inflammatory flavonoids and cinnamic acids, both are anti-cancer phytonutrients. Fiber in a pear will keep you regular. Plus, pears may decrease your risk of type 2 diabetes.1 cup raw: calories: 51; fat: 0g; sodium: 0mg; carbs: 13g [4g dietary fiber, 9g sugars]; protein: 1g; Vitamin A: 0%; Vitamin C: 8%; Calcium: 0%; Iron: 0%. Storage: Pears, which need to be ripened, can be put in a sealed plastic bag with a couple of ripe bananas at room temperature. Ripe pears may be refrigerated until ready to eat it.

Peppers: Bell peppers are a great source of vitamin C and carotenoids. A recent study with peppers showed a lower risk of developing gastric cancer and esophageal cancer when consumed. 1 cup chopped, raw: calories: 30; fat: 0g; sodium: 4mg; carbs: 7g [3g dietary fiber, 4g sugars]; protein: 1g; Vitamin A: 11%; Vitamin C: 200%; Calcium: 1%; Iron: 3%. Storage: If placed in a plastic bag, peppers will last a week in the refrigerator.

Phytonutrients: Nutrients only derived from plants.

Pomegranates: Superfood! Pomegranates are a good source of dietary fibers, both soluble and insoluble, which aid in healthy bowel movements and smooth digestion. They are recommended for weight loss and lowering your cholesterol. Being loaded with vitamin C, they can boost your immune system and improve circulation and offer protection against cancers, such as prostate cancer. They have punicalagin and tannins which are effective in reducing heart disease. Regular consumption has been found to be effective against diabetes and lymphoma. Pomegranates contain many vital B-complex vitamins, folates, pyridoxine and vitamin K, plus, essential minerals like calcium, copper, potassium, and manganese. 1 raw: calories: 234; fat: 3g; sodium: 8mg; carbs: 53g [11g dietary fiber, 39g sugars]; protein: 5g; Vitamin A: 0%; Vitamin C: 48%; Calcium: 3%; Iron: 5%.

Potatoes: Potatoes may get a bad rap but they are packed with more potassium than bananas, broccoli or spinach. They are a super source of vitamin C and contain the vitamin B6 and a small amount of thiamine, riboflavin, folate, magnesium, phosphorous, iron, and zinc. 1 large, raw w/ skin: calories: 284; fat: 0g; sodium: 22mg; carbs: 68g [8g dietary fiber, 3g sugars]; protein: 7g; Vitamin A: 0%; Vitamin C: 121%; Calcium: 4%; Iron: 16%. Storage: Cool (45°F to 50°F) humid (but not wet) surroundings. Refrigeration can turn the starch in potatoes to sugar and may tend to darken when cooked.

Quinoa: (pronounced KEEN-wah) has the highest nutritional profile and cooks the fastest of all grains. It is an extremely *high energy* grain and has been grown and consumed for about 8,000 years on the high plains of the Andes Mountains in South America. The Incas were able to run such long distances at such a high altitude because of this powerful grain. Contains: all eight amino acids to make it a complete protein; has a protein content equal to milk; high in B vitamins, iron, zinc, potassium, calcium, and vitamin E; gluten-free; easy to digest; ideal food for endurance; strengthens the kidneys, heart, and lungs. 1 cup raw: calories: 222; fat: 4g; sodium: 13mg; carbs: 39g [5g dietary fiber]; protein: 8g; Vitamin A: 0%; Vitamin C: 0%; Calcium: 3%; Iron: 15%.

Rhodiola: Rhodiola is an herb. It is an antioxidant believed to help with mental fog, physical performance, stress and fatigue, plus, it enhances your immune system.

Spinach: Superfood! Rich in omega-3 fatty acids. Fights against things like breast and skin cancer. 1 cup raw: calories: 7; fat: 0g; sodium: 24mg; carbs: 1g [1g dietary fiber, 0g sugars]; protein: 1g; Vitamin A: 56%; Vitamin C: 14%; Calcium: 3%; Iron: 5%. Storage: Remove bad leaves, trim off stems, wash thoroughly in cold water. Repeat until grit is gone. Spin dry or drain well. Loosely wrap with paper towel and put in a plastic bag. Place in the refrigerator, spinach only lasts a few days.

Swiss Chard: Contains phytonutrients benefiting your body's blood sugar-regulating system, which may provide special benefits for those diagnosed with diabetes. Chard contains a healthy amount of fiber and has a good amount of protein. It's an excellent source of vitamin C, vitamin E, vitamin A and the minerals manganese and zinc. Swiss chard also has antioxidants. With a good amount of calcium, magnesium and vitamin K, it provides great bone health. 1 cup raw: calories: 7; fat: 0g; sodium: 77mg; carbs: 1g [1g dietary fiber, 0g sugars]; protein: 1g; Vitamin A: 44%; Vitamin C: 18%; Calcium: 2%; Iron: 4%. Storage: Do not rinse, wrap it up in plastic wrap and it can last for up to two days in the refrigerator.

Tomatoes: Tomatoes have been known to reduce the risk of heart disease, this is due to their antioxidants and their ability to help regulate fat in your bloodstream. Tomatoes have been shown to decrease LDL cholesterol and decrease triglyceride levels (sugar in your blood). They support bone health. They say tomatoes may lower risk of prostate cancer in men along with non-small cell lung cancer, pancreatic cancer and breast cancer. Diets that include tomatoes may reduce the risk of neurological diseases, such as Alzheimer's disease, shown in multiple studies. Plus, a regular diet of consuming tomatoes may lower risk of obesity. 1 cup raw: calories: 27; fat: 0g; sodium: 7mg; carbs: 6g [2g dietary fiber, 4g sugars]; protein: 1g; Vitamin A: 25%; Vitamin C: 32%; Calcium: 1%; Iron: 2%. Storage: Keep at room temp until ripened. Once ripened, they will last for two to three days. Tomatoes can be refrigerated in veggie bin for approximately one week. Try to avoid refrigerating because they can lose their flavor.

Walnuts: Great source of omega-3 fatty acids, reduces the risk for heart disease/plaque build-up in the arteries, lowers bad cholesterol, rich in fiber, B & E vitamins and magnesium, rich source of plant-based protein and reduces triglycerides (fat in the blood). 1 cup chopped: calories: 765; fat: 76g; sodium: 2mg; carbs: 16g [8g dietary fiber, 3g sugars]; protein: 18g; Vitamin A: 0%; Vitamin C: 3%; Calcium: 11%; Iron: 19%.

Wheat Grass: Creates energy, full of amino acids benefiting muscle building. 4g: calories: 15; fat: 0g; sodium: 0mg; carbs: 2g [1g dietary fiber, 0g sugars]; protein: 1g; Vitamin A: 30%; Vitamin C: 12%; Calcium: 1%; Iron: 44%.

10

IN A NUTSHELL— OVERCOMING POSSIBLE CHALLENGES

In a nutshell, let me provide you with a list of challenges you may be combating against and what foods to reach for to help with the matter.

*Having **trouble pooping?*** Reach for: apples, artichokes, beans, cabbage, carrots, chili peppers, flaxseed, honey, mangoes, oats/oatmeal, peaches, pineapple, prunes, wheat germ, wheat bran and yogurt.

*Lovely subject, but **they do happen: hemorrhoids?*** When you're having trouble with pooping you may end up with hemorrhoids from all of the stress of pushing while sitting on the porcelain throne (the toilet). Help combat hemorrhoids by having some: beans, cabbage and peaches.

*Having trouble with **diarrhea?*** Help stop it by eating: apples, bananas, pineapples and rice.

*Wanting to prevent **colds or the flu?*** Gobble up the following: bananas, cantaloupe, dark-leafy greens, goji berries, oranges and pineapples.

*Want to improve **your lung capacity while exerting yourself out on the ice?*** Here are some things you should be picking up from the store and eating more of: apples, oranges and quinoa.

*Concerned about your **joints?*** Eat apples! Apples help cushion your joints from all of the impact they endure.

*What about your **precious bones, too?*** Promote strong bones by eating: bananas, beets, broccoli, cauliflower, green beans, kale, mushrooms, pineapple, sweet potatoes, swiss chard, tomatoes and yogurt.

*Having trouble with **seeing the puck and your teammates?*** I would first suggest you see your ophthalmologist (your eye doctor) to get your vision checked. You may hear your parents or grandparents complain about poor night vision when they drive at night . . . well, let's help you keep that issue at bay for as long as you can by indulging in the following: apricots, broccoli, cantaloupe, carrots, grapes, kale and sweet potatoes.

*Feeling a little **stressed out?*** Have some strawberries and get active, get out on the ice and check someone! Be sure to be getting the proper amount of sleep for *you.*

*Family **heart issues?*** Stop the vicious cycle by enjoying foods like: apples, bananas, beets, blueberries, broccoli, cabbage, carrots, cherries, chestnuts, fish, grapefruits, grapes, green tea, lemons, limes, olive oil, onions, oranges, peanuts, rice, strawberries and tomatoes.

Family history of **high blood pressure?** Reach for: apricots, avocados, bananas, beets, broccoli, cantaloupes, chestnuts, figs, garlic, lemons, limes, mushrooms, oatmeal and watermelon.

Zits? **Dull skin?** May I suggest: avocados, coconut oil, goji berries, guavas, lemons, limes, mangoes, melons, oats/oatmeal, olive oil and water. Yep, once again, water! Water! Water! Water!

What about **issues with stabilizing your blood sugar?** Are you sometimes as mean as a bear? Could be your blood sugar level is simply low. Let's talk about the things which can help your blood sugar levels: artichokes, bananas, beans, blueberries, brown rice, coconut oil, oatmeal and swiss chard.

Want to **live to be a happy and healthy 100 year old?** *Me, too!* You can begin the possibility by eating the foods which help you slow the aging process: apricots, beets, cherries and prunes. Plus, cook with coconut oil.

Do any of **your elders have Alzheimer's?** Please try to prevent from getting it yourself by stocking up on: apricots, cherries, lettuce, mangoes, oranges and tomatoes.

Want to try your best to combat against getting **cancer?** Let's consider enjoying the following foods to help combat it: apricots, beans, beets, blueberries, broccoli, cabbage, cantaloupe, carrots, cherries, chestnuts, chili peppers, figs, fish, garlic, grapes, green tea, lemons, limes, mangoes, mushrooms, oats/oatmeal, olive oil, onions, oranges, peaches, peanuts, rice, strawberries, sweet potatoes, tomatoes, walnuts, water, wheat germ and wheat bran.

Family history of **diabetes?** Consider battling against it with the following: almonds, avocados, flaxseed, oats/oatmeal, oranges, pears, pomegranates, swiss chard and using olive oil.

Okay, forget about food for a moment. Here are some added helpful tips:

Injuries: When treating an injury think *R.I.C.E.*

R = Rest
I = Ice* (20 minutes 4x/day; with a thin cloth)
C = Compression (for support, but not too tight)
E = Elevate (keep injured area above heart to reduce blood flow and swelling to the area).

> **Ice first 48 hours to help with pain/swelling. Once swelling is gone, you may apply heat.*

Proper stretching. To avoid a hamstring pull, place your foot up on a chair and bend forward at the hip, do not bounce; switch and do the other side. To avoid groin pull, lie on your back and do the butterfly stretch. Place a ball between your knees and squeeze. To avoid ACL tears/strains, strengthen quadriceps muscles (front of thigh).

Gatorade vs. Water. When you're on the ice for more than 60 minutes it is okay to grab a sports drink to alleviate dehydration and to replenish minerals and electrolytes. Avoid caffeine, which can bring on dehydration.

For **growing pains,** take a hot shower or bath and eat pineapple (natural pain reliever).

Being fit! Benefits of *being fit.* Better energy, better mood, improved self-esteem and better overall health. It's that simple. Be proud of your fit physique and SHINE!

SLEEP—Did you know that your cells regenerate when you sleep? Sleep deprivation can wreak havoc on the immune system. Please try to get at least 7-9 hours of sleep each night so you won't get run down, and make it a healthy habit to go to bed and rise at roughly the same time each day/night.

SWEAT—Want to know how to speed up your metabolism and improve your immune system? Simply sweat! When you sweat, your body releases toxins, allowing it to produce more white blood cells. Your white blood cells are the "army men" of your immune system. Result, less days sick in bed, which means less hockey games and practices missed. You're doing it not only for yourself but for your team!

Neti Pot—What is a Neti Pot? When is it best to use one? It's a lead-free, ceramic pot which you fill with distilled saline water and you pour the water through your nasal passages. This process helps assist the body by cleaning out any bacteria, excess mucus, allergens, and other irritants from the cilia (little, hair-like structures) of your nose and it helps to soothe dry nasal passages.

Primary Foods . . . Eating great nibbles can be a real pleasure but food really should be secondary to the more important things in life. Consider for a moment if we thought about our relationships, our career, our spiritual being and our physical being as our primary foods. Try that on for size and watch how food becomes a treat, not a threat to our well being. *(Want to work on your primary foods? Contact me via my website at www.NHLhealthcoach.com)*.

Happy and Healthy! Create a healthier, happy, balanced life. Say "please", "thank you" and "hello" with a smile; be kind, thoughtful and generous; count your blessings; ask "What good things happened today?"; play music; sing; dance; laugh; de-junk and de-clutter; go outside; soak up the sun; take a deep breath; turn off the TV and open a book; slow down; and be positive. *Create healthy habits* and watch your life change for the better; your achievements will be many.

Your body is your temple. Make what you put into your body as important as the effort you put in while on the ice. *Listen to your body.* If you have cravings, your body is telling you the nutrients which are missing.

Cholesterol. Know your numbers. Your HDL, also known as your good cholesterol, should be greater than 60. Your LDL, known as the bad cholesterol, should be less than 100. Your optimal Total Cholesterol should be less than 200.

Read the labels. When reading labels on packaged goods, try to avoid foods which have more than five ingredients listed under the "Ingredients" list. Also, if you can't pronounce an ingredient put the product back on the shelf and forget about it. Please don't put it into your body.

Worry or Laugh? Which sounds like a better time? How about thinking of it this way: Worry is like a stray dog, feed it and it'll stay around. My grandfather used to say, "Worry is a debt you may never have to pay." And, my grandma used to say, "Worrying doesn't change the outcome." How about instead of worrying you find someone who makes you laugh and never let go. It will add years to your life.

What are your top three *values?* Write your top three down today and live by your values. Here are a few you may consider:

- faith
- family
- love
- integrity
- authenticity
- wealth
- happiness
- adventure
- friends

Say "thank you" to your mom/dad. It is a privilege to play ice hockey. Take a moment today to thank the one who put you in your first pair of ice hockey skates.

AVOID these simple carbs: Soda, can- dy, desserts, white bread, baked treats, coffee with sugar and syrups, ice cream and anything made with white sugar.

Benefits of eating your *greens.* Purifies blood; prevents cancer; improves circulation, as well as, the functioning of your kidneys, liver and gall bladder; reduces mucus/congestion; promotes intestinal flora, strengthens immune system; energy; lifts spirit, less depression. Greens to try: bok choy, cabbage, kale, collards, watercress, mustard greens, broccoli rabe, arugula, endive, chicory, mesclun, wild greens, spinach, Swiss chard and beet greens.

If you *need to* **gain weight,** eat more calories at each meal and eat more often (5-6 times per day). Try to drink a quart of milk (fat-free/skim) every day.

Simple meal: Roast, grill or bake pork tenderloins, salmon, tuna steaks, bison, white fish, turkey and/or chicken breasts. Service with brown rice or quinoa and add any vegetable you have a craving for. Enjoy with a tall glass of fat-free/skim milk.

Something to think about: Stop for a moment and give this some thought. Where would you like your health to be three months from now? How about six months from now? What obstacles, challenges and struggles do you have with regard to diet/lifestyle? What are five things you LOVE about your life? In what areas of your life would you like to find more balance with regard to family, friends, school, work, sports, education, finances, health, physical activity, home environment, home cooking, social life, joy or your spirituality?

Baby Steps. By taking small steps to a happier, healthier lifestyle, you will soon begin to experience an amazing transformation. We are not looking for perfection, but progress in the right direction for your best life ever! What is it that you are currently experiencing? What is your present state? Where is your attention? What are your emotions? What is the intended positive outcome of your current experience? What does someone have to believe about your current state? What beliefs are you currently holding dear? Are your beliefs needing to be updated? Tweaked a little? What if you could change your present state; would you?

What is your desired state? Where would you like to be mentally, physically, emotionally, spiritually a month from now, three months from now, six months or a year from now?

If you are ready to begin to take baby steps into understanding nutrition, not only for your body but for your mind and soul, please reach out to me for private, one-on-one coaching.

Years ago, I attended the Institute of Integrative Nutrition (IIN) to become a board certified holistic health coach. At IIN we learned more than 100 dietary food therapies from teachers including Dr. Andrew Weil, Director of the Arizona Center for Integrative Medicine; Dr. Deepak Chopra, leader in the field of mind-body medicine; Dr. David Katz, Director of Yale University's Prevention Research Center; Dr. Walter Willett, Chair of Nutrition at Harvard University; and many other leading researchers and nutrition authorities. However, what I loved the most from my experience at IIN was the founder, Joshua Rosenthal's, approach to holistic health. Holistic meaning the "whole person." Joshua explained to us that our primary food isn't food, our primary foods are our relationships, our physical being, our spiritual being and our careers. He taught us practical lifestyle coaching methods. It made total sense to me but I needed to go deeper, I needed more.

A few years ago, I attended IIN's mega conference in Long Beach, California, where over 5,000 health coaches from all over the world gathered together with one GIGANTIC desire. We all were there to figure out how we could change the world. How could we make it a happier, healthier world? You know how? By helping one individual at a time. There will never be enough health coaches; there are too many people to help. If you find becoming a health coach of interest to you, reach out to me and I'll share with you, in great detail, my journey of becoming a health coach.

11

RECOMMENDED FOODS & BEVERAGES

Take this list to the grocery store with you and try some things you've never tried before. You know I'm a huge fan of only one-ingredient foods and nothing in a package but if you're buying something that comes in a package, please be sure to read the label. Here are seven simple rules:

Rule #1

No more than 10g of sugar, preferably < 5 g per serving

Rule #2

No more than 600g of sodium per serving

Rule #3

No saturated, no trans fats, no partially hydrogenated oil

Rule #4

If there's the suffix "ose" (i.e. gluc*ose*) it's added sugars

Rule #5

No more than five ingredients in the ingredient list

Rule #6

If you can't pronounce an ingredient put it back on the shelf

Rule #7

If your grandparents wouldn't recognize it as a food, don't buy it

BEVERAGES:

- Water
- Coconut water
- Kombucha
- Lemonade/green lemonade
- V8 (low sodium)
- Homemade smoothies or *Naked* fruit smoothies
  - » Milk (2% or non-fat/fat-free/skim; FairLife™ is a fabulous brand with 50% more protein and less sugar)
  - » Decaf coffee (no more than 3 cups a day; 1 cup for children)
  - » Decaf hot tea (no more than 6 cups a day; 1 cup for children)
  - » Decaf iced coffee (no more than 3 cups a day; 1

cup for children)

» Decaf iced tea (no more than 6 cups a day; 1 cup
for children)

» Regular coffee** (no more than 2 cups a day; not
recommended for children)

» Regular hot tea** (no more than 2 cups a day; not
recommended for children)

» Regular iced coffee** (no more than 2 cups a day;
not recommended for children)

» Regular iced tea** (no more than 2 cups a day; not
recommended for children)

NOTE: If you like to add cream to your coffee or tea, please
use only *regular* half-and-half, do not use fat-free. Why? Take
and compare labels next time you're at the grocery store. If
you need to add sweetener use Raw Sugar, though if you're
looking to scale back on calories try Truvia or Stevia.

*** Do not consume after lunch, as it can interrupt sleep*

FRUITS:

- Fresh or frozen fruit only (steer away from canned)
- Apples
- Bananas
- Blueberries
- Blackberries
- Cantaloupe
- Cherries
- Grapefruit (as long as it doesn't conflict with
medications)
- Grapes (green and red)
- Honeydew melon

- Strawberries
- Raspberries
- Peaches
- Pears
- Tomatoes
- Watermelon (minimal)
- Pineapple (minimal)
- Plums
- Apricots
- Kiwi
- Mango
- Papaya
- Oranges, tangerines and Clementines
- Nectarines

VEGETABLES:

- Fresh or frozen vegetables only (steer clear of canned)
- Artichoke
- Asparagus
- Bamboo shoots
- Beets
- Broccoli
- Brussels sprouts
- Cabbage (green, bok choy, Chinese)
- Carrots
- Cauliflower
- Celery
- Cucumber
- Daikon
- Eggplant
- Greens (collard, kale, mustard, turnip)

- Green beans
- Hearts of palm
- Jicama
- Leeks
- Mushrooms
- Okra
- Onions
- Pea pods
- Peppers
- Radishes
- Rutabaga
- Salad greens (chicory, endive, escarole, lettuce, romaine, spinach, arugula, radicchio, watercress)
- Squash
- Sugar snap peas
- Sweet potatoes
- Swiss chard
- Tomatoes (really it's a fruit, but I'm putting in here, too, because I don't want you to miss it)
- Turnips
- Water chestnuts
- Zucchini

- Lentils
- Legumes
- Dried beans (lima, black and pinto; no canned)
- Dried peas (split and black-eyed)
- Nuts (tiny bowl serving, 2 x day)
- Olives (tiny bowl serving, 1 x day)

OILS & SPICES:

- Coconut oil
- Olive oil (PAM Olive Oil Cooking Spray)
- Regular, low-sodium butter (use sparingly)
- Garlic
- Pepper
- Sea Salt (per American Diabetics Association; unless you have thyroid issues then use iodized salt)

Note: Some people try to use salt substitutes instead of table salt. Some substitutes are high in potassium, which could be harmful. Check with your physician before using salt substitutes and make sure they won't interfere with another medical condition or your medications if you take them. http://www. diabetes.org/food-and-fitness/food/what-can-i-eat/cutting-back-on-sodium.html

FISH/SEAFOOD:

- catfish
- cod
- flounder
- haddock
- halibut
- herring
- orange roughy
- salmon
- tilapia
- trout
- tuna
- sardines
- clams
- crab

- lobster
- scallops
- shrimp
- oysters

POULTRY/MEAT

- Chicken
- Turkey
- Cornish hen
- Eggs/Egg Whites
- Beef tenderloin
- Lamb
- Organ meats: heart, kidney, liver
- Veal
- Pork
- Buffalo/Bison
- Ostrich
- Venison

12

RECIPES

GREEN DREAM SMOOTHIE™

Ingredients:
Handful of spinach
1/2 of an avocado
1 banana
5-6 chunks of pineapple
1 scoop of Skoop™
8-16 oz of water
6 ice cubs

Directions:
Load the ingredients into your Vitamix, or blender, and let 'er rip! You can add more water or ice, play around with it and find your happy medium. This is a great way to get two servings of veggies and two servings of fruit into your diet for the day.

Where to get SkoopTM? For $10 off, visit:
http://coachloves.healthyskoop.com

BOUNCING BISCUITS™
(NO BAKING REQUIRED!)

Ingredients:

1 cup of oatmeal
1/2 of natural peanut butter
1 cup of sweetened coconut flakes
1/3 cup of agave nectar
1/4 cup of chia seeds
1/2 cup of mini, dark-chocolate chips
1 tsp vanilla

Directions:

In a large mixing bowl combine all of the above ingredients and mix well. Cover the bowl and place in the refrigerator overnight or keep refrigerated for a minimum of four hours. Remove from refrigerator and by hand roll into 1″ balls. NOTE: Bouncing Biscuits will hold for one week in the fridge when put in an airtight container.

Experience incredible energy with Bouncing Biscuits™!

GREEN LEMONADE

Ingredients:
2 handfuls of spinach & kale
1 green apple
½ cucumber
1/4 of a peeled lemon
1 scoop of Skoop™
32 oz of water
6 ice cubes

Directions:
Load all ingredients into Vitamix (or blender). Start on low, increasing speed until highest speed is reached. Let blend for a minute or two. Drink 16 oz. and reserve the other 16 oz. for mid-morning snack or afternoon snack. Drink it down with a straw.

Where to get Skoop™? For $10 off, visit:
http://coachloves.healthyskoop.com

HOMEMADE ENERGY DRINK

Ingredients:
16 oz of water
1/4 cup of juice (such as orange, lemon, lime or pineapple)
pinch of sea salt

Directions:
Mix together—ENJOY! The natural way to replenish your electrolytes.

SLAPSHOT SMOOTHIE™

Ingredients:
4 oz. Greek, organic yogurt
handful spinach
½-cup blueberries
1 apple
1 banana
1 scoop of Skoop™
16 oz water, ice.

Directions:
Blend all ingredients for a minute or two (add or subtract the amount of water and ice to your liking). Drink with a straw and feel the goodness going down!

Nutritional Facts: Cal: 262; Fat: .3g; Cholesterol: 0mg; Sodium: 75.7mg; Potassium: 849.9mg; Carbs: 58.1g [9.3 g dietary/37.5g sugars]; Protein: 13g; Vitamin A: 59.3%; Vitamin C: 39%; Calcium: 21%; Iron: 8.5%

Where to get Skoop™? For $10 off, visit: http://coachloves.healthyskoop.com

THE BENJAMIN BOWL

Ingredients:
1 can of organic, low sodium black beans
1 pouch of Seeds of Change® certified organic
    quinoa & brown rice
1 cup of organic salsa
1 teaspoon of minced garlic
Optional: tortillas

Directions:
Rinse black beans well and place into a sauce pan along with the salsa and garlic over medium heat, stirring on occasion. When the beans are fully cooked, pop the quinoa and rice pouch into the microwave for 60-90 seconds. Mix all ingredients in individual bowls or if you'd prefer a burrito, throw the mixture into your tortilla(s) and serve.

This is the healthy alternative for when you're Jones'ing for something from Chipotle.

TRAVIS HOWE OATMEAL DELIGHT

Ingredients:
1-4 cups steel-cut oatmeal
1-4 cups water or almond milk
1-4 peeled and diced apples
Cinnamon

Directions:
In a CrockPot® stir in oatmeal and water or almond milk in equal portions, such as one cup of oatmeal to one cup of water or almond milk. The amount of oatmeal you choose to use depends upon the amount of servings you want to make. Next, peel and dice your apple(s) and place on top of your oatmeal mixture and sprinkle with cinnamon.

In a CrockPot® cook for approximately 7 ½ hours on the LOW setting. (NOTE: time can vary depending on various crock pots and the temperature in which they cook).

How awesome is that to wake up to? It is like eating apple pie in the morning! Makes your mouth water doesn't it? I can smell it "baking" now.

FRESH TURKEY BREAST

Ingredients:
1 fresh or frozen turkey breast
1/2 cup of water
1 teaspoon of thyme
1 teaspoon of sage

Directions:
Let the frozen turkey breast sit overnight in the refrigerator. You can either prepare in the morning or in the evening depending upon if you want it for dinner or to use for things like fresh turkey sandwiches. Rinse turkey breast and place in CrockPot® with water and sprinkle thyme and sage over breast. Set on low and cook for 7-9 hours depending upon the number of pounds.

Remove from CrockPot® and carefully remove netting. Serve with brown rice and/or quinoa and your favorite vegetables for dinner or slice and use for sandwiches, etc.

13

JOURNALING

Keeping a journal or diary can be very helpful for your evolution—for your personal growth. As I have suggested over and over again, keep track of how foods and beverages affect you. How did you feel physically and emotionally? Here are some things you can make note of:

- When?
- What food(s)?
- What was your hunger/thirst level?
- Where were you when you ate?
- What was the current situation (at home or on-the-go)?
- How much did you have?
- What time of the day did you eat?
- How was the food/beverage prepared?

Here are some things you may be experiencing either physically or emotionally:

PHYSICAL SIGNS:

- Poor concentration
- Headaches
- Stomach aches
- Muscle cramps/weakness
- Coughing
- Fatigue
- Insomnia (can't sleep)
- Restlessness
- Shakiness
- Clear, white eyes
- Stamina
- Improved energy
- Peaceful sleep
- Great focus
- Alertness
- Glowing complexion

EMOTIONS:

- Anxious
- Bored
- Frightened/scared
- Angry/mad/irritable/agitated
- Sad/depressed
- Restless/hyper
- Confident
- Excited/enthusiastic
- Energized
- Humorous
- Happy
- Calm/relaxed/easygoing/patient

Keeping a food journal is designed to be informative and helpful for keeping track of which foods/beverages do or do not work for you as an individual.

Another great reason to journal is if you are experiencing challenges in your life. Writing emotions and thoughts out on paper will help you "work things out." It is also a lot of fun to look back and see what you were thinking about and what you were doing during certain times in your life, so save your journals. There are times when you will want to sit back and reflect where you've been, what you've endured and be able to look at how far you've come. Someday, you may choose to share your personal discoveries and accomplishments with your significant other or even your children. This will provide them a glimpse into your soul.

However, when you're writing in your journal/diary, trust that no one is reading it. Be open and honest with yourself. You may never care to share such intimate details of your life, but there may come a time when sharing your personal findings/struggles/challenges, etc., may be just what you need in order to see a relationship grow.

Just like praying, there is no particular way in which to write in your journal—there's no right or wrong. Just simply begin to write. Write and write and write some more. You won't believe what unfolds when you do. Capture memories which you never want to forget. Write down your dreams. When your dreams come true celebrate them! Take note of your feelings, of your thoughts and emotions.

14

SETTING GOALS & ACHIEVING THEM

I would like to share with you some of the goals I set for myself and how I accomplished each and every one of them. I am an *entrepreneur* . . . that "title" for me was *unbelievable* a few years ago but here I am today a proud business owner. I am a motivational speaker. I am an author. I set out to help others change their lives for the better and my clients are strutting around in their new improved bodies, happier and healthier than they ever have been in their lives.

A couple of years ago when I was saying good night to my son, I said to him, "I just want to thank you and your sister for being so understanding, loving and supportive with mom's journey with building her business. I know I'm traveling a lot and have to spend time with clients, which I would normally be spending with you two, but please continue to be patient and trust that mom will be successful." My son's response to me, "It's your time to shine, Mom." And, that, folks, is the name of one of my programs: "It's Your Time to Shine"!

It is important to invest in our relationships, education, career, home(s), etc., but it's critical that you invest in yourself. What do you want to do when you grow up? Who do you want to be? Where do you want to be? What is your greatest desire? Envision yourself exactly where you want to be and with whom. Think positive thoughts and push out any negative ones.

You can be and do *anything* you desire. You need to believe in yourself, have faith and trust. The universe wants this for you. Now go out there and get it! I believe in you. I am proud of you. *The puck stops here . . .*

RESOURCES

Acai:
http://www.mayoclinic.org/healthy-living/nu-
trition-and-healthy-eating/expert-answers/acai/
faq-20057794

Banana:
Source: http://www.karenstan.net/ Read More: http://www.
natureknows.org/2013/10/after-reading-this-youll-never-
look-at.html

Brown Rice:
1 "Brown Rice." *WHFoods.* www.whfoods.com 2 *The
Government of the Hong Kong Special Administrative
Region.* http://www.cfs.gov.hk

Carbs:
http://www.nutritionmd.org/nutrition_tips/nutrition_tips_un-
derstand_foods/carbs_versus.html

Cauliflower:
http://articles.mercola.com/sites/articles/archive/2014/02/22/
cauliflower-health-benefits.aspx

Chia Seeds:
http://www.webmd.com/diet/features/truth-about-chia

Coconut Oil:
The Surprising Health Benefits of Coconut Oil

By Pina LoGiudice ND, LAc, Siobhan Bleakney, ND, and Peter Bongiorno ND, LAc Co-Medical Directors of Inner Source Health in New York

Flaxseed:
www.webmd.com/diet/features/benefits-of-flaxseed

Goji Berries:
http://www.huffingtonpost.ca/2014/03/28/goji-berry-benefits-_n_5044948.html

GMOs:
http://action.greenamerica.org/p/salsa/web/common/public/signup?signup_page_KEY=7626&gclid=CMyuqZTl7L0CFecWMgod42YAmQ

Ingredients to Avoid:
http://health.yahoo.net/experts/eatthis/8-ingredients-you-never-want-see-nutrition-labelDiary:

[1] MyPyramid.gov—Inside The Pyramid—How much food from the milk group is needed daily? February 3, 2011. Available at: http://www.mypyramid.gov/pyramid/milk_amount.aspx#.

[2] FAQ—Dairy. The Weston A. Price Foundation. Available at: http://www.westonaprice.org/faq/784-faq-dairy?qh=YTo5Ont pOjA7czozOiJyYXciO2k6MTtzOjc6InJhd25lc3MiO2k6Mjtz OjQ6Im1pbGsiO2k6MztzOjc6Im1pbGtpbmciO2k6NDtzOj U6Im1pbGtzIjtpOjU7czo2OiJtaWxrZWQiO2k6NjtzOjg6I m1pbGtpbmdzIjtpOjc7czo2OiJnbWlsayciO2k6ODtzO jg6InJhdyBtaWxrIjt9.

[3] The New Four Food Groups. Physicians Committee for Responsible Medicine. Available at: http://www.pcrm.org/health/veginfo/vsk/4foodgroups.pdf.

[4] Release No. 0059.10. United States Department of Agriculture. February 10, 2010. Available at: http://www.usda.gov/wps/portal/usda/usdahome?contentidonly=true&contentid=2010/02/0059.xml.

[5] Why Does Organic Milk Last So Much Longer Than Regular Milk? Scientific American. June 6, 2008. Available at: http://www.scientificamerican.com/article.cfm?id=experts-organic-milk-lasts-longer.

[6] The Dangers of Raw Milk: Unpasteurized Milk Can Pose a Serious Health Risk US Food and Drug Administration. May 5, 2011. Available at: http://www.fda.gov/Food/ResourcesForYou/Consumers/ucm079516.htm

[7] Calcium and Milk – What's Best for Your Bones and Health? The Nutrition Source. Harvard School of Public Health. Available at: http://www.hsph.harvard.edu/nutritionsource/what-should-you-eat/calcium-full-story/index.html.

[8] Dhiman, T. R., G. R. Anand, et al. Conjugated Linoleic Acid Content of Milk from Cows Fed Different Diets. 1999. J Dairy Sci 82(10): 2146-56. Available at: http://www.journalofdairyscience.org/article/S0022-0302%2899%2975458-5/abstract.

[9] Vitamin D and Chronic Disease – Your Nutrition Questions Answered. The Nutrition Source. Harvard School of Public Health. Available at: http://www.hsph.harvard.edu/nutritionsource/questions/vitamin-d-and-chronic-disease/.

[10] Lactose Intolerance: Information for Health Care Providers. National Institutes of Health. January 2006. Available at: http://www.nichd.nih.gov/publications/pubs/upload/NICHD_MM_Lactose_FS.pdf.

[11] Mitigating the Greenhouse Gas Balance of Ruminant Production Systems Through Carbon Sequestration in Grasslands. Food and Agriculture Organization. Vol 11-2010; p 121. Available at: http://www.fao.org/docrep/013/i1880e/i1880e05.pdf.

[12] Greenhouse Gas Emissions from the Dairy Sector: A Life Cycle Assessment. Food and Agriculture Organization of the United Nations. 2010. Available at: http://www.fao.org/docrep/012/k7930e/k7930e00.pdf.

Lignans:
Lignans linked to healthier, thinner women: Study
By Stephen Daniells, 06-Feb-2009

Women with increased intake of lignans, and subsequently levels of metabolites in the blood, tend to have lower BMIs and total body fat mass, says a new study from Canada.

http://www.nutraingredients.com/Research/Lignans-linked-to-healthier-thinner-women-Study

Nutritional Tidbits:
www.nutritiondata.self.com
www.whfoods.com

Oatmeal:
http://www.whfoods.com/genpage.php?tname=foodspice&dbid=54

Rhodiola:
http://www.drweil.com/drw/u/QAA400399/Rhodiola-for-What-Ails-You.html

Soda:
http://www.healthenlightenment.com/soda.shtml

http://www.howmuchisit.org/
how-much-does-coke-drink-cost/

Sodium:
http://www.nlm.nih.gov/medlineplus/ency/article/002415.
htm

http://healthyeating.sfgate.com/average-daily-sodium-teen-age-boy-3466.html

Sugar:
http://www.bjcschooloutreach.org/addingitupsugar

ABOUT ROXANNE TUOMELA

Roxanne is a Board Certified Holistic Health Coach, Master in TCM (Transformational Coaching Method) and member of AADP (American Association of Drugless Practitioners). She is the founder/owner of NHL Health Coach where she works with individuals one-on-one and with teams in group programs; you can also find her as a guest speaker/coach at hockey camps around the country. Her passion for happy and healthy living began over 30 years ago when she lost all of her family members in a ten year span, except for her older brother and a handful of cousins. She is determined to live a long, healthy life so that her own children do not have to endure the loss she had to experience at a young age. Roxanne is on a quest to become a vibrant and active centenarian.

So her journey began, not only with a goal to live to be 100, but because she was also sick and tired of dull hair, brittle nails, feeling lethargic, and stuffing her overweight body into skinny jeans with a bloated belly.

Roxanne knows firsthand about life-threatening food allergies and intolerances. Developing an allergy to shellfish landed her in the emergency room where she was told, "You might not make it to the ER in time, the next time." For years, she dealt with skin rashes and hives before uncovering what foods caused her personal trouble.

Roxanne is the proud mother of two children, a son in high school and a daughter in middle school, both of whom are active in sports. Her son has been playing ice hockey for over ten years.

Roxanne enjoys the building of great leaders on and off ice. There simply isn't enough time for coaches to cover all bases. She says, "Leave the high-speed skating development, stick handling, off-ice strength training and rules of the game to the coaches and but ask me to help with the critical growth and development of each individual player mentally and physically, as a whole, through nutrition and transformational coaching."

It was at the Institute for Integrative Nutrition where Roxanne was trained in more than one hundred dietary theories and studied a variety of practical lifestyle coaching methods with some of the world's top health and wellness experts. Her teachers included Dr. Andrew Weil, Director of the Arizona Center for Integrative Medicine; Dr. Deepak Chopra, leader in the field of mind-body medicine; Dr. David Katz, Director of Yale University's Prevention Research Center; Dr. Walter Willett, Chair of Nutrition at Harvard University; and many other leading researchers and nutrition authorities.

Roxanne received her Master Certification in TCM from Holistic MBA. With her transformational coaching methods her clients are able to uncover beliefs and behavioral patterns which stem from their past experiences. Such discoveries allow her clients to tweak or update their beliefs, thus, changing their behavioral patterns, with the end result being clients who reach their desired state.

Her coaching skills/methods are the tools she uses to help hockey players become remarkable team players and effective leaders not only in sports but in life.

For further information on how to work with Roxanne send an email to NHLhealthcoach@gmail.com.

Learn more about Roxanne at www.NHLhealthcoach.com

FREE "THE PUCK OF LIFE"

Take a few minutes to download your free copy of my Puck of Life exercise tool. Take this opportunity to discover where there may be some imbalance in your life.

www.NHLhealthcoach.com/puckoflife

CONNECT WITH ROXANNE

Websites
Coaching for Hockey Players/Teams:
www.NHLhealthcoach.com

Coaching for Individuals/Groups:
www.healthcoachkiely.com

Coaching for Rapid Recovery/Life Transition:
www.AGL.Club

10-Day Transformational Cleanse:
www.mypurium.com/AGLclub

FREE Strategy Session!
If you would like the opportunity to have a free strategy session with Roxanne, visit:
https://my.timedriver.com/1P5QR

Social Media
Instagram: NHLhealthcoach
Twitter: NHLhealthcoach
Facebook: Roxanne Tuomela Kiely

Direct
301-325-0287

Email
NHLhealthcoach@gmail.com

ROXANNE'S FAVORITES

Non-Profit Organizations:
Stop Concussions (Keith Primeau)
www.stopconcussions.com

Charities Challenge (Gary Westlund)
www.charitieschallenge.org

Training:
Legacy Global Sports
Selects Hockey (Travis Howe/Mitch Larnerd)
www.legacyglobalsports.com

Off-Ice Stickhandling (Lance Pitlick)
www.sweethockeycoach.com

FHIT Hockey (Garrett Gruenke)
www.fhithockey.com

MAP Hockey
www.maphockey.net

Mouthguards:
Impact Mouthguards
www.impactmouthguards.com

Hockey Shops:
Dave's Sport Shop
www.davessportshop.net

Lettermen Sports
www.lettermensports.com

Hockey Central
www.hockeycentralinc.com

Protein Powder:
B-Strong by SkoopTM
http://coachloves.heathyskoop.com

Photography:
Divine Photography
www.divinephoto.net

CPSIA information can be obtained
at www.ICGtesting.com
Printed in the USA
BVHW01s0137281217
503690BV00001B/33/P